Genetics and Society

There was an unprecedented growth in knowledge about the genetic basis of disease in the last decades of the twentieth century. *Genetics and Society* looks at the social circumstances of these developments and their implications for the future. Using fascinating and cutting edge examples throughout, Anne Kerr casts a critical eye over topics as diverse as:

- the past, present and future of genetic knowledge and technologies;
- the place of professionals, patients, families and publics in genetic research and service provision;
- the social and cultural construction of genes and disease.

Each chapter begins with a summary and ends with suggestions for further reading, making the book accessible to a wide readership. *Genetics and Society* will be essential reading for anybody with an interest in the social aspects of genetics.

Anne Kerr is lecturer in the Sociology department at the University of York, UK.

Genetics and Society

A sociology of disease

Anne Kerr

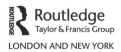

Routledge
Taylor & Francis Group

LONDON AND NEW YORK

First published 2004
by Routledge
11 New Fetter Lane, London EC4P 4EE

Simultaneously published in the USA and Canada
by Routledge
29 West 35th Street, New York, NY 10001

Routledge is an imprint of the Taylor & Francis Group

Typeset in Garamond by
Newgen Imaging Systems (P) Ltd, Chennai, India
Printed and bound in Great Britain by
MPG Books Ltd, Bodmin

British Library Cataloguing in Publication Data
A catalogue record for this book is available from the British Library

Library of Congress Cataloging in Publication Data
 Genetics and society: a sociology of disease / Anne Kerr. – 1st ed.
  p. cm.
 Includes bibliographical references and index.
  1. Medical genetics – Social aspects. 2. Genetics – Social
aspects. I. Title.
 RB155.K477 2004
 362.196′042–dc22   2004001266

ISBN 0–415–30081–9 (hbk)
ISBN 0–415–30082–7 (pbk)

Contents

List of boxes   viii
Acknowledgements   ix

1 Introduction   1

Summary 1
Introduction 1
Why this book now? 3
Themes and chapters 9
Past, present and future 10
Patients, professionals and publics 11
Knowledge, practice and things 12

2 Past   15

Summary 15
Introduction 16
Surveillance, coercion and voluntarism 18
Prevention 22
Reductionism 24
Commerce, governance and expertise 28
Contemporary debates about eugenics 30
Conclusion 36
Further reading 37

3 Discovery   38

Summary 38
Introduction 38
The discovery discourse 43
Knowledge, practice and things 45
Commercialization 46

Governance 50
Expert relations 53
Defining disease 56
Conclusion 62
Further reading 62

4   **Reproduction**   64

Summary 64
Introduction 64
Reproductive choices 66
Down's syndrome screening in the United Kingdom 74
Conclusion 82
Further reading 83

5   **Patients**   84

Summary 84
Introduction 84
The psychosocial approach 86
Biography narratives 89
Risk and responsibility 94
Conclusion 101
Further reading 102

6   **Biobanks**   103

Summary 103
Introduction 103
Informed consent 106
Privacy and confidentiality 111
Commercialization and governance 116
Conclusion 121
Further reading 122

7   **Publics**   123

Summary 123
Introduction 123
Public opinion 125
Lay knowledge 132
Active citizenship 134
Constructing citizens and publics 138
Conclusion 142
Further reading 142

8 Futures 143

Summary 143
Introduction 143
Policy-speak 145
Public bioethics 148
Biomedicine 154
Mass media 156
Conclusion 160
Further reading 160

9 Conclusion 161

Introduction 161
Past, present and future 162
Patients, professionals and publics 163
Knowledge, practice and things 165
Researching genetics and society 167

Glossary 170
Notes 174
Bibliography 175
Index 189

Boxes

2.1   Eugenics and genetics   16
3.1   Discovering the Charcot-Marie-Tooth and distal spinal
muscular atrophy gene – the National Human Genome
Research Institute's version   40
3.2   CF History Project – discovering CF   58
4.1   CF History Project – interview with two CF specialists:
clinician working with adults with CF and molecular geneticist   67
4.2   'Transformations in Genetic Subjecthood' ESRC Project
– Interview, 2002   69
4.3   OSCAR   76
4.4   The Integrated Test   77
4.5   The Antenatal Screening subgroup of the UK National
Screening Committee   78
6.1   Insurance and employment   110
6.2   Nationhood   117
7.1   Attitudinal groups from the Office of Science and
Technology and The Wellcome Trust (2000)   126
7.2   MORI genetics poll shows public's confusion,
12 March 2000   129
7.3   Increasing public support for controversial technologies   130

Acknowledgements

I would like to thank The Wellcome Trust History of Medicine Programme and the Economic and Social Research Council for financial support during the period of writing. I would also like to thank the National Institute of Health, USA, the Office of Science and Technology and The Wellcome Trust for permission to reproduce material herein. Thanks also to Mari Shullaw for commissioning this book when she was at Routledge and to Gerhard Boomgaarden for seeing the project through to completion. Sarah Cunningham-Burley, Klaus Hoeyer, Richard Tutton, Mandy Rees, Steve Yearley and Clare Williams have given valuable feedback on various draft chapters, for which I am very grateful. Special thanks are due to Gillian Robinson for compiling the bibliography and copyediting the manuscript. Finally, thanks to my family, especially Brian Woods, for their encouragement and support throughout the period of writing.

1 Introduction

Summary

In this chapter, I begin by outlining some of the key developments in the study, diagnosis and treatment of genetic diseases, and their social implications. I highlight five specific aspects of genetics and society that I think ought to be investigated:

1   The fascination with what is new and different about contemporary genetic technologies and knowledge, and the corresponding tendency to ignore not so new technologies and caricature the links between the past and the present.
2   The focus upon the transformative effects of genetic knowledge and technologies on patients and publics, rather than the social conditions which give rise to their development and implementation.
3   The prevailing emphasis upon patients' individual choices in much of the discussion about genetics and society, despite considerable evidence that their choices can never be autonomous or based upon neutral information and are but one part of the relationships between genetics and society.
4   The considerable attention, paid by governments, scientists and social researchers, to the public understanding of genetics, and their views on how genetics should be controlled and regulated: attention which nevertheless fails to translate into a democratization of decision-making in this area.
5   The tendency to take genes for granted where the relationships between genetics and society are concerned.

I go on to outline the three main themes that are explored in the book: past, present and future; patients, professionals and publics; and knowledge, practice and things; and give a synopsis of the chapters that follow.

Introduction

There was an unprecedented growth in research into the genetic basis of disease in the last decades of the twentieth century. A range of genetic tests is now available to people with family histories of genetic disorders. Mostly, these are prenatal tests, which can identify and terminate affected foetuses. Couples using assisted conception techniques, such as in vitro fertilization (IVF), can also access genetic tests to identify unaffected embryos for implantation in the woman's womb. Genetic tests are now available to so-called high-risk populations as well. For example, in some areas, pregnant women are offered genetic screening for disorders like cystic fibrosis. Presymptomatic tests are also available to some people with family histories of genetic diseases that occur later in life, such as Huntington's disease. Other such tests are also available for genes involved in rare hereditary forms of more common diseases such as breast cancer. Tests for genes related to nutrition have also been developed and marketed directly to the public as an aid to health and lifestyle planning.

Although relatively small numbers of people, often with quite specific concerns, are using these tests, they are part of a much larger programme of research into the genetic basis of disease. The sequencing of the human genome involved a massive international research project known as the Human Genome Project (HGP). Other researchers plan to collect DNA from populations, as large as four million people in the case of UK Biobank, in an effort to understand the genetic basis of common diseases like cancer or heart disease. Alongside these flagship projects, a range of smaller-scale studies are being conducted into the genetics of single gene disorders, the development of gene therapies which target faulty genes and the proteins they produce, and pharmacogenomic treatments tailored to respond to an individual's genetic make-up. The knowledge and techniques of modern molecular and clinical genetics are also being used in stem cell and embryo research projects, with the aim of preventing and treating serious diseases.

These developments have not taken place in a social or cultural vacuum. The scientific and clinical practices of genetics and associated fields of enquiry have developed in an era where professionals are subject to considerable public scrutiny by the media and a range of campaigning organizations, including disability rights, pro-life and animal rights activists. Patient groups are also increasingly involved in shaping the research agendas of the scientists and clinicians who treat them. The commercial interests in much modern day genetics have been a source of particular tension between companies, governments, activists, patients and professionals, especially when it comes to the issue of patenting genes, and the implications of these practices for research and product development. A range of ethical quandaries exists alongside these commercial concerns, particularly when it comes to parents' rights to choose the characteristics of their children and the aim of perfect health that seem to be the goals of modern genetics. The legacy of eugenics inevitably overshadows these debates, particularly the history of coercion and intolerance of diversity. Yet, most people would argue that choice and tolerance of difference reign supreme in this era of late modernity, except, perhaps, for those who cannot afford to participate in the consumer society.

Social scientists have studied these developments in genetics and society as they have occurred, concentrating in particular upon the experiences of patients, especially pregnant women, the representation of genetics in popular culture, and the public understanding of genetics. Others have looked at the social and ethical aspects of new or emergent technologies, such as biobanks. Scholars have paid less specific attention to the practices of government or professionals, although there are some notable exceptions, particularly when it comes to laboratory practice, or the links between commercial organizations and the development and implementation of regulations at national and international levels. Yet, it is scholars from other disciplines that have come to dominate public discussion about these issues, notably bioethicists who have concentrated upon the ethics of the choices thrown up by these new technologies. Scientific and medical professionals are also publicly reflexive about the work in which they are involved.

Why this book now?

The scale of contemporary genetic research and technology aimed at disease prevention, its considerable social and ethical implications, and the need for a greater sociological presence in contemporary discussions about genetics and disease are three reasons to focus upon the sociology of genetic disease in this book about genetics and society. A synthesis of the various strands of social research into the social and ethical aspects of genetic disease will also be useful for students and scholars interested in the subject. However, I am also motivated to write such a book by another set of more specific concerns.

The first relates to the focus upon new technologies that not only characterizes much of the public discourse about genetics, but also dominates much of the social research in this area. On a superficial level, this taste for novelty is understandable, particularly in popular culture. Uncharted territory is also likely to stimulate researchers' interests, particularly when this involves working alongside scientists and clinicians as their knowledge and technologies develop. However, individual researcher's interests do not drive this focus upon the new. Other social and political arrangements also foster research in new areas, at the expense of traditional, long-standing or apparently mundane aspects of science and medicine. In recent years, research funding organizations, governmental bodies and commercial organizations have increasingly focused upon the social implications of new or emergent medical technologies. They often present this as an effort to anticipate and manage public concerns about new technologies. Noteworthy research programmes that address the social and ethical dimensions of the biosciences, at the behest of a range of corporate, medical and social research agencies, make this clear. For example, the UK Economic and Social Research Council's (ESRC) Innovative Health Technologies Programme (co-funded by the Medical Research Council and GlaxoSmithKline)[1] and the Wellcome Trust's Medicine in Society Programme, both stress, in the words of the Wellcome Trust, the 'breathtaking' pace of discovery in the life sciences and the 'unprecedented questions' this poses for society.[2] Thus social research on science or medicine often focuses upon the social implications of new technologies, looking at their clinical applications, or public perceptions of their worth, for example. Researchers are also encouraged by funding agencies to identify and work with so-called user groups, so that their results can influence policy and practice.

Although this type of work is valuable in many respects, it does have a number of side effects that are rather less welcome. Researchers that are oriented towards helping scientists to implement new technologies more successfully, tend not to be able to question the ways in which these types of technologies emerge and develop over the long term. A broad historical perspective is lost when speculation about the future dominates. In the area of genetics, this is particularly problematic, given the history of eugenics. As I shall argue in Chapter 2, and throughout this book, a great deal of the contemporary discussions about genetics involve boundaries between the past and the present. This often involves caricatures of the past, as a time when eugenicists, in collaboration with brutal dictators, abused science in the interests of population improvement. Today's geneticists are widely represented as applying knowledge in the fight against disease, offering people more choices and opportunities to improve their health and that of their offspring. We pay little attention to the links between the past and the present. Indeed, when comparisons between the past and the present are drawn, they are often dismissed as extreme forms of anti-science.

When social researchers foreground what is new about these technologies, and focus upon their social impact, they risk perpetuating these distinctions between past and present, and reinforcing the rationale of enlightenment and individualism in the process. It is therefore important that we understand how certain developments are represented as new, at the same time as we explore their historical context. In order to understand genetics and society, we also need to look at what is not so new as well as what is apparently new about genetics. We need to look at the ways in which social relations have shaped the development and implementation of the knowledge and technology of genetics, rather than focusing upon the impact of technology on society. The place of social research on genetics in the promotion and support of genetic science and medicine also requires consideration.

This brings me to the second and related trend that I wish to address in this book: the prevailing emphasis on transformation in modern societies, and the presentation of new genetic technologies as an important driving force behind these changes. As Andrew Webster, the director of the ESRC's Innovative Health Technologies Programme has noted,

> contemporary innovations are not simply extending the medical repertoire and the instruments available to it but are *transforming* it. In addition, these innovations are changing our understanding of health, illness and disease, so redefining health, medicine and the body.
>
> (Webster, 2002: 446)

A significant portion of the sociological literature in this area foregrounds the transformative effects of new genetic technologies on the patients who use them. This is sometimes linked to an explicit rejection of comparisons between the past and the present. Nikolas Rose and Paul Rabinow eschew comparisons between the new genetics and eugenics (Rabinow, 1996, 1999; Rose, 1999, 2002) on the grounds that, in the words of Rose: 'our very biological life itself has entered the domain of decision and choice' (Rose, 2001: 22, see also Rabinow, 1996). Rose argues that a contemporary 'logic of control' is enacted through the ethics of the genetic counselling session and the registries and databases of the information society. Individual susceptibility and individual choice are at the core of these logics, alongside complex and fragmentary notion of genes and their functions (Rose, 2001). This suggests that people can, to a certain extent, choose their own genetic futures, subverting and reinterpreting genetic information rather than simply following doctor's orders.

Other social theorists have also highlighted the potential of these technologies to transform social relationships more broadly. Ulrich Beck's work on the risk society develops these themes, focusing upon the ways in which technologies manufacture risks that have thrown doubt on the projects of modernity (Beck, 1993, 1995). Consumer choice and large-scale technological hazards are said to undermine established social stratification and notions of scientific progress and, in so doing, enable alternative social arrangements based on 'dialogic democracy' (Giddens, 1990) and 'technologies of doubt' (Beck, 1993).

This focus upon transformation seems to have many of the problems of the focus upon the new. Foregrounding the transformative effects of technologies takes attention away from the social circumstances in which they are developed, and the extent to which they reinforce old cultural values and social arrangements, rather than introduce new ones. This is especially true in the area of reproductive genetic screening which many argue reflects particularly negative views of disabilities like Down's syndrome (Hubbard, 1997; Lippman, 1999b; Williams *et al.*, 2002a). Associating broad shifts in democratic arrangements to technological developments and their attendant risks also seems to neglect the many ways in which modern liberal democracies have adapted to contain public unease without necessarily opening up moral or political dialogue to different voices and experiences. As Carole Smith has argued, moral thinking has in many ways been hijacked by dominant discourses of 'rights talk', which reduces everything to a question of people's rights and duties and stifles any open and radical discussion of morality (Smith, 2002). I have also argued, with Sarah Cunningham-Burley, that the institutions of modern science can easily adapt to counter any threats to their authority that might come from the public at large by co-ordinating consultation exercises with a democratic gloss (Kerr and Cunningham-Burley, 2000).

This raises questions about how different groups of people make sense of these new genetic technologies by focusing upon their transformative potential. For government and professionals, foregrounding transformation might be a way of bolstering public support for these new technologies by delineating them from the past. Transformation is also a powerful commercial discourse that underlines the novelty and desirability of new genetic treatments and diagnostic technologies, highlighting their powers to predict and cure genetic disorders. For others with a stake in social change, new clinical services may be seen as having the potential to empower patients and publics, not only to plan their own life choices based upon genetic information, but also to organize in order to challenge the risks posed by these new technologies. Other groups opposed to new genetic technologies explicitly reject this focus upon broad social and cultural transformations, because their arguments rest upon the identification of strong and enduring parallels with the past. However, they may still invest considerable transformative power within these technologies: to oppress, rather than to liberate, the people who use them.

These different approaches to the issue of transformation raise a number of questions that I will explore in the course of this book. How are the technologies and knowledge of contemporary genetics framed in relation to the past and the future, by people with an interest in this area? What are the key differences in how particular technologies and their social effects are presented and interpreted by different people? How flexible are the boundaries that they erect between past, present and future in these discourses?

This takes me onto the third area that I wish to explore in more detail in this book: the emphasis upon individual choice in the arguments of proponents and critics of genetics alike, as well as those who analyse their arguments. This relates to the discussion earlier, as individual choice is one of the key ways in which present practices tend to be delineated from the past. We need to explore when and how these types of distinctions are drawn, and to what effect. We also need to explore the ways in which discussions of the future flow from and reinforce particular preoccupations with choice in the contemporary era.

The predominant focus in much of the current research on genetics is upon patients' experiences of making choices about genetic tests. This is especially true in the area of reproductive genetics, where numerous research studies have been conducted into people's experience of being offered testing or screening, their decision to proceed or decline, and the role of counselling therein (see Clarke, 1991; Marteau *et al.*, 1993; Green, 1995; Johanson *et al.*, 2000; Marteau and Dormandy, 2001). Although most of these authors convincingly demonstrate that women's choices are far from autonomous or based purely on objective information, the rhetoric of informed choice remains in much of the medical and bioethical literature in this area. Why?

There also appears to be a real imbalance in the ways in which we study individual choice in relation to genetic technologies. We focus upon the individual choices of patients but not the choices of the people who developed and implemented these technologies in the first place. This is hardly surprising in the more applied types of health service research that are explicitly focused upon improving service provision; but even in the more sociologically oriented work on patients' experiences, professional practices remain largely in the shadows. It is therefore important to throw some light on these matters if we are to understand genetics and society in its fullest sense. We also need to think about how people come to be categorized as patients in the first place, and whether it is always appropriate to analyse their experiences in this way.

When patients are not the focus, publics often take their place. Perhaps surprisingly in an area that is so closely associated with individuals' clinical encounters, there is a considerable body of work on the public understanding of genetics. This is largely driven by government officials' and scientific professionals' concerns about the lack of public trust in their work. They are keen to know about the public understanding of genetics and what influences it, so that they can act upon the results to clarify misapprehensions and foster public trust. Much of this work is rather pedestrian and conservative: focused upon what the public do not know about the technicalities of genetics. However, consultation and research exercises are increasingly concerned with public perceptions of scientific practice in its broadest sense, and have begun to take seriously public concerns about accountability and transparency in policy-making in this area. This is particularly apparent in areas of new technological development like biobanking. Does this institutional reflexivity signal professionals' newfound responsiveness to public concerns? Are members of the public influencing policy-making in meaningful ways? Who are the public, anyway?

Another boundary between past and present which can often be found when genetics is discussed involves a distinction between old-fashioned notions of genes as fixed determinants of disease and behaviour, and new, contemporary notions of genes as complex, interactive and contested entities. The death of genetic determinism is widely accepted by all but the most trenchant critics of the new genetics. These definitions of genes and their newfound malleability clearly require analysis, along the lines I have already suggested. Who constructs these divisions between past and present? How are old genes different from new genes? How do ideas about genes and ideas about disease and deviance shape each other?

At the same time, genes are widely held to be real, natural phenomena and therefore not worthy of social enquiry. Indeed, there is tremendous hostility to the idea that genes or other natural phenomena might be socially constructed. As Bruno Latour has noted, scientists often assume that people who want to investigate the social aspects of nature are trying to show that natural objects are the repository of social factors, rather than incontrovertible objective entities of nature. They are concerned that this devalues the enterprise of science, by turning it into just another belief system, like religion or magic (Latour, 2000). Social scientists tend to share this wariness of looking at natural sciences and nature because they want to be scientific about society (not nature). This involves explaining how social factors and functions cause behaviour, attitudes, perceptions or discourses. Thus genes remain a fact of nature for most social scientists with an interest in genetics and society.

We also tend to think of genes as the bedrock of genetic disease: genetic diseases occur because of faulty genes, so if you find the gene you can move towards preventing or treating the disease. This is 'science-lite': a parable for popular consumption, promoted by scientists through press releases and popular science. Anyone who has actually worked in this area will tell you that the links between genes and diseases are far more complex. However, apart from a few sociologists and anthropologists of science and technology, social scientists are not terribly interested in these issues. We might raise questions about the level of the genetic contribution of common, complex disorders like heart disease or cancer, because we want to make our own points about the social factors determining disease. However, the processes involved in identifying genes or their social equivalents and using them to understand disease are left largely unquestioned. This, again, is difficult territory, because asking questions about the social aspects of genes might lead people to think that you doubt the existence of diseases, many of which are distressing and painful for the families that they affect. This means the genetic basis of genetic disease is largely taken for granted in most analyses of genetics and society.

The idea that genes form the bedrock of genetic disease also dominates sociological explanations of people's experiences of genetic disease. Postmodernism notwithstanding, social scientists often treat people's biological, or in this case genetic, deficiencies as the mainstay of their experiences of living with disease. For example, researchers might chart people's experiences or perspectives on their lives according to the progression of their disease. This is reflected in medical sociology theories that frame illness in relation to biographical disruption (Bury, 1982) or 'loss of self' (Charmaz, 1983). When they are applied to genetic diseases, these types of explanations privilege genes as causal factors in people's illness and experience of that illness, paying less attention to the myriad relations that shape how people come to articulate their experience of disease.

I want to question what genes are and what role they play in people's experiences and definitions of disease. This means that they must be understood within the context of laboratory and clinical practice, but I do not intend to expose them as social rather than natural entities. As Latour has long argued, studying the social construction of things like genes or disease is not a matter of swapping a materialist explanation for a social one. Rather it is about giving non-human actors their proper place in sociology. This type of sociology of genetic disease is not premised upon the identification of the social factors that determine how genes are constructed, just as it does not involve the identification of social factors that determine how geneticists or people affected by genetic diseases behave. We can investigate the sociology of genetics without treating society as a source of explanation for what genes are, or how people behave. Instead, we can think about how social order comes about through the association of people and things such as genes and diseases. Genes do not represent or contain social factors any more than people do.

Both are hybrid actors – at once social and material entities – entwined in assemblies or networks of relationships. People and things are influenced by their relationships with their surroundings, but they are also unpredictable, difficult to control, and obdurate: what they are changes as we study them. Their actions do not simply reflect something out there called 'society'. Instead, we should focus upon the ways in which people and things create social order through their interactions with each other.

Exploring the social construction of genes is not about showing how genes are really just reflections of society. We need to think about how they are produced by scientists, clinicians, patients and non-human actors, including the things that are extracted from people's bodies in the process of studying genes. This means looking at how explanations for what counts as a gene or a genetic disease take form, and are shaped by the practices of the people who are working with them. We can also explore how scientists and clinicians come to identify things that they call genes, what shapes these processes, and how this relates to their ideas about the disease they are studying. Diseases and genes are made from bits of bodies, as well as the people associated with them and the techniques used to diagnose and treat them. Their meanings change over time and in different settings. A historical perspective on these processes provides rich insights into how genetics is both transforming and transformative.

This also applies to how we account for people's experience of genetic disease. As disability activists and scholars from disability studies have pointed out, representations of people's experiences are political. The image of people suffering from, or at the mercy of, their genetic disease, not only promotes work designed to cure them, but could also be taken to implicitly support more controversial preventative methods, such as selective abortion. For many disabled people, this smacks of eugenics. For others, especially those affected by rare disorders, it is an important way of drawing attention to their situation, and of generating resources for better services and treatments. This suggests that we also need to be careful to think about how people's experiences of genetic disease come to be represented in different ways, and how the meanings of disease, just like the meanings of genes, are co-produced by different actors – human and non-human.

Themes and chapters

These issues can be divided into three main themes which structure the remainder of this book: past, present and future; professionals, patients and publics; and knowledge, practice and things. I have divided this book into eight main chapters (in addition to this introductory chapter and the conclusion, Chapter 9). Each chapter covers aspects of all three themes, but focuses upon one theme in particular. Past, present and future is the main theme addressed in Chapter 2, 'Past' and in Chapter 8, 'Future'. Professionals, patients and publics is the main theme addressed in Chapter 5, Patients' and in Chapter 7, 'Publics'. Knowledge, practice and things is the main theme addressed in Chapter 3, 'Discovery', in Chapter 4, 'Reproduction', and in Chapter 6, 'Biobanks'. This means that the chapters can be read as stand alone case studies for people interested in particular aspects of genetics and society, but can also be read as a series of discussions that build towards an overall analysis of genetics and society based upon these three principal themes.

Past, present and future

Different constructions of the past and the future, and the ways in which technology, knowledge, patients, professionals and publics are represented by their authors, are explored in Chapters 2 and 8, respectively.

Chapter 2 concerns the ways in which contemporary genetics is framed in relation to the past by a range of social actors. I will begin by considering the types of boundaries that supporters of genetics tend to draw between eugenics and genetics, and explore these throughout the chapter. This builds upon a range of historical studies of eugenics and genetics, and previous work on professionals' discourses about eugenics (Kerr *et al.*, 1998a; Kerr and Shakespeare, 2002). I will argue that eugenics cannot be dismissed as a thing of the past, largely because it remains a powerful notion in contemporary discussions about genetics. However, I will also note that eugenics is very flexible – it is associated with a range of discourses and practices. Genetics and eugenics have interacted with each other in important respects, but not in others. The way in which people account for these changes varies depending upon their support for or opposition to particular technologies or policies, their experience or otherwise of genetic disease, and their relationships with other consumers, companies, experts and policy-makers.

Important discourses such as individual choice and social progress are also examined in relation to constructions of the past, the present and the future in Chapters 4, 5 and 6. These chapters address particular developments in genetic research and practice, so discourses about their benefits often involve boundaries between the past and the present, and the invocation of cures and treatments for patients of the future. These chapters focus upon what I consider to be more established developments in genetic research and services, rather than other areas of research which are less clearly established in the laboratory, or technologies which have not yet had a significant impact upon clinical practice. I focus upon the discovery of genes involved in disease, reproductive technologies, particularly screening, and biobank research. These areas of genetics have also been well researched by social scientists, which makes them good case studies.

I focus more specifically on emergent technologies in Chapter 8. This looks at future discourses around gene therapy, genetic enhancement and cloning. I have chosen to package these new technologies together in a chapter about future discourses, rather than to examine their potential to change clinical practice in its own right. This is largely because I think that deconstructing the discourse of future potential is more interesting than speculating about how these technologies may or may not be implemented in the clinic, especially since they are a long way from being used in this way. A range of actors are involved in these discussions, including policy-makers, bioethicists, scientists and journalists. The way in which they frame the benefits and risks of these imagined futures depends upon how they are placed in the present, in relation to the different groups involved with genetic research and clinical practice, including funding and regulatory agencies, corporations and patient organization. It also depends upon their relationship to the material involved in this research, like genes or cell lines, and especially controversial actors such as embryos. I explore the different discourses of future potential and future risks that these actors create, and consider their implications for how we conceptualize our ownership and control of technological development.

Patients, professionals and publics

In addition to understanding how the past and the future are constructed in contemporary genetics and society, we also need to consider the location of patients, families, publics and professionals. This involves looking at how these various groups are represented in genetic research and commentaries about the social aspects of genetics, including how they position themselves in these processes. Two key chapters are devoted to examining these subject positions.

In Chapter 5, I will explore the various ways in which patients and families are represented in a range of analyses of patients' experiences. I will show that the psychosocial approach of medical professionals tends to pathologize people's experiences, and to root them in an underlying biological deficiency. This makes people with direct experience of genetic disease into patients and ignores the other identities they might assume in their daily lives. This can also happen where parents of children with genetic diseases, or members of families considered to be at high risk of particular genetic diseases, are concerned. Although work in medical sociology has challenged this emphasis upon the biological body, it can also reinforce a sense in which patients and their families are the victims of their biology, by focusing upon how they cope with their illness. Other work has looked at people's experience of genetic disease within a much broader context. This has shown that the identity of 'patient' is not hegemonic, and that it means different things to different people.

This discussion develops some similar points made earlier in Chapter 4 concerning women's experiences of reproductive genetic testing and screening. Here I draw attention to the various ways in which these technologies fit into women's life worlds, and how this depends upon a range of different relationships with their unborn child, families, professionals, communities and so on. However, the clinical encounter allows little time for an exploration of these networks and how they might shape any decision regarding testing. Instead, the identity of patient is foregrounded.

I pick up similar themes in Chapter 6 on biobanks, when I consider how research subjects are not only constructed as passive patients by proxy, but also as active health consumers. Large scale biobank research has also been subject to considerable public scrutiny, because of its very public nature, in the sense of the numbers of people it involves, and its implications for the public health. This has meant that a range of competing subject positions also exist along-side that of patient or consumer, particularly the position of citizen. It has also meant that professionals have been especially reflexive about their own subject positions in relation to the research and clinical applications of biobanks, and that they have actively constructed ethical personas as part of this process.

In Chapter 7, I will look much more closely at how the public are constructed in discussions about genetics and society, notably in terms of their ignorance or lack of trust. I will focus upon social research into public opinion, understanding and perceptions of genetics and its social context, and consider how these various constructions of the public are translated in the governance of genetics. This chapter is especially influenced by my own research interests in this area, particularly the work of two research projects in which I have been involved.[3] Drawing on some recent findings, I will explore the ways research in this area constructs positions for research subjects to occupy, such as 'authentic citizen'. I will also consider how research subjects resist or subvert these types of positioning, in favour of their own expressions of expertise. The imagery of the public nevertheless remains an important aspect of professional and policy communities' rationales for action.

Knowledge, practice and things

The ways in which bodies, instruments and people co-produce genetics are the main issues discussed under this theme. These issues are explicitly addressed in Chapter 3, 'Discovery.' In this chapter, I deconstruct the discourse of discovery in genetics and link it to the social and economic context in which genetic research takes place. Drawing on a range of studies of laboratory and professional practice, and ongoing research into the history of cystic fibrosis,[4] I consider the ways in which commercialism, governance, and professional relationships shape the focus and aims of genetic research and the very processes by which things get to be called 'discoveries'. I am especially interested in how notions of genes and ideas about diseases interact, and the difficulties of mapping genetic information onto explanations of disease, and vice versa. The recalcitrance of things is an important aspect of these processes, as are the relationships between and among scientists, clinicians and patients. However, I will also explore how this contingency and messiness comes to be deleted from particular representations of the discovery process, notably the institutional press release.

Chapter 4 is about reproductive technologies, particularly genetic screening. I begin with an exploration of the ways in which choice and responsibility are presented in discussions about various kinds of reproductive genetic technologies. I then move on to consider the social context in which these technologies emerge and are sustained. These technologies result from complex webs of relationships between professionals, patients, policy-makers and the instruments and substances involved in the testing process. However, women's choices have little impact on the design and implementation of these technologies. Professionals articulate rather than simply facilitate consumer demand. Although screening programmes can become entrenched in health care systems, and women's choices are often circumscribed by the clinical context in which they take place, the diversity of the experiences and relationships shaping their decision mean that reproductive choice can be both enabling and constraining.

Chapter 6 is focused upon the governance of genetic research in the case of biobanking. Although this chapter is about regulating the production of genetic knowledge rather than the production process in its own right, the two are intrinsically linked via professional practice. Biobank research depends upon the collection, storage and acceptable use of DNA, which involves setting up and enacting specific protocols of informed consent and confidentiality. This chapter explores the ways in which these protocols are presented in the professional literature, and what this tells us about professional practice in this area. I also explore what happens when donation occurs, and the ways in which information and consent are negotiated in the process. I stress the flexible principles and practices at stake in this area, and the tensions around the rights and responsibilities of the different actors that shape them. I also explore the different ways in which professionals manage these tensions as they proceed with research.

In Chapter 9, the book concludes by considering what these seven substantive chapters have added to our understanding of genetic disease and its social context. Returning to the questions raised earlier in this introductory chapter, I consider the ways in which the various actors involved with research and technologies which are focused upon the prevention of genetic disease, and the constructions of their risks and benefits, are both heterogeneous and flexible. However, I am also keen to find some common threads between the actors, technologies and discourses that genetic diseases involve, both in terms of the past, present and future, and in terms of the relationships between people, things and discourses that they involve. Contested notions of social progress and tensions around individual rights and societal responsibilities seem to be particularly salient across all of these domains. I end by reflecting upon the ways in which research into genetics and society might develop and add to our understanding of these processes. I make a case for more research into the social and physical arrangements that shape the development of not so new genetic technologies, and query the role of social research which is oriented to future technologies in supporting their emergence. I also question the preoccupation with patients and publics, and the perpetuation of narrow and unreflexive framings of their subject positions in contemporary research. Case rather than subject oriented social research might mediate against these problems by providing a more rounded picture of how a range of actors are positioned in relation to particular forms of knowledge and technology, although this also has its drawbacks. On a more positive note, I recognize that some of the most innovative work in this area involves close collaborations between scientists, clinicians and social researchers, particularly ethnographic studies of laboratory and clinical practice. Although the danger of being dazzled by science and medicine is ever present, social researchers working in these environments have given us important insights into how genetic knowledge and technologies are developed and applied. The difficulties of ethical approval notwithstanding, this might be a fruitful model for understanding how genetic knowledge and technology translates in other domains beyond the laboratory and the clinic, to the home, the workplace and the institutions of contemporary governance.

2　Past

Summary

In this chapter, I begin by considering some of the dichotomies between genetics and eugenics that are the subject of debates about the risks and benefits of contemporary genetic knowledge and technologies. These include divisions between

- the objectivity and neutrality of modern day genetics, as opposed to the subjectivity and biases of eugenics;
- the holistic and complex understanding of contemporary genetics as opposed to the reductionist and simplistic understandings of the past;
- the focus upon disease today, as opposed to the focus on deviancy in the past;
- and the contemporary emphasis upon individual choice, in contrast to the coercive population policies of the past.

I then explore to what extent these dichotomies hold up when the history of eugenics, from the early part of the twentieth century to the postwar era. I will argue that eugenics has always been associated with a variety of ideologies and practices, in the past and the present. At times, genetic knowledge has been mobilized in support of certain eugenic ideas, and a range of professional and academics with an interest in medicine and science have tried to put these ideas into practice. However, others associated with genetics have challenged the place of eugenics in clinical practice, and the ideas about genetic fitness and racial supremacy with which we have come to associate eugenics.

Eugenics continues to be a topic of vigorous debate in contemporary discussions about genetic technologies. The commercialism of genetics and its links with genetics is especially contested. I argue that the dynamics of expertise and governance are both reflected in and shape these contemporary discussions. I conclude by noting the flexibility of the dichotomies that I outlined at the beginning of the chapter. Consumers, companies, experts and policy-makers form various alliances in support or opposition to particular genetic developments, be they technological or regulatory, and tailor their discourses of eugenics accordingly.

Introduction

Eugenics is an important topic in professional and popular debates about the social and ethical implications of new genetic technologies such as prenatal diagnosis, gene therapy and cloning. Critics, often from the disability right movement, argue that these technologies have been designed to eradicate disability, and improve the population, not by overt coercion, but in the guise of health choices. Proponents of genetics respond by arguing that their accusers have an exaggerated sense of the technical capabilities and political powers of scientists and doctors. They distinguish genetics from the outdated and discredited ideology of eugenics. For example, Tom Wilkie (a science journalist) has argued that in its hey day (the 1920s and 1930s) eugenics involved concern about the 'gene pool' of the future [white] race which took precedence over the autonomy and rights of the individual, or indeed the unborn child and that 'a better understanding of human and general genetics gradually undermined [this] eugenicist position' (Wilkie, 1993: 164).

We can broadly simplify these characterizations of genetics and eugenics in Box 2.1.

These dichotomies suggest that eugenics is not a contemporary phenomenon: it has been superseded by the neutral, objective knowledge of genetics that has done away with biased knowledge, and misapplication outside the legitimate realm of medicine. In contrast to eugenics, today's genetics has the interests of the individual at its core; it provides people with more choices about their health and their families' health, as part of a modern health care system. This also casts contemporary geneticists as responsible, legitimate professionals, serving the interests of their clientele, offering them choices, treating disease and providing them with information, which is their right. These characterizations key into contemporary cultural emphasis upon the sanctity of the individual, the valorization of choice, and the benefits of medical knowledge.

Box 2.1 Eugenics and genetics

Eugenics	*Genetics*
Past – Pre-Second World War	Present – Post Second World War
Ideology (i.e. biased)	Science (i.e. objective)
Reductionist	Balanced
Abuse of knowledge	Pure knowledge properly applied
Populations	Individuals
Coercion	Choice
State	Market
Social deviance	Disease

However, these dichotomies are highly contested in a climate where medical science is not universally recognized as neutral and objective. There are growing calls for deeper and more widespread regulation of scientists' and doctors' activities, and a deep suspicion about the use of medical information for surveillance and social control. Activists from the disability movement are often highly critical of genetic science and technology, drawing parallels between the history of the Nazi holocaust and compulsory sterilization and today's termination of genetically defective foetuses. They have argued that abortion laws that sanction late terminations on the grounds of serious handicap are examples of modern eugenic policy (Bailey, 1996). As Rock has argued,

> Disabled people know only too well they are not welcomed in society, but the active promotion of abortion on the grounds of disability and determining that euthanasia is a viable proposition for the disabled foetus/child – is fascism.
>
> (Rock, 1996: 124)

For critics of contemporary genetics the lines between past and present, ideology and knowledge, coercion and choice, are a charade.

This makes the history of genetics, particularly human genetics one of the most politically charged of the modern sciences. Geneticists, and mainstream historians, tend to favour linear, internalist histories of the subject, where the focus is upon famous scientific milestones, decontextualized from the cultural and political contexts of the time (see Super, 1992; Brock, 2002 as examples; Kerr *et al.*, 1998a, for an analysis of geneticists' discourse about eugenics in interviews). Historians from a more sociological tradition focus instead upon the social relation that shaped, and were shaped by, scientific knowledge and practice. In the case of genetics, this inevitably leads to discussion of the troubled relationship between eugenics and the development of genetics. Historians and sociologists in this genre have challenged simplistic definitions of eugenics, as a form of pseudo-science or compulsory sterilization. Rather, they have shown the many and varied associations between eugenics and genetics, up to and including the development of the Human Genome Project and molecular genetic tests. As Diane Paul argues that, 'it is ... highly improbable that ... canned histories, with their total contempt for the past, will promote a critical perspective of current developments in biomedicine' (Paul, 1992: 664).

In this chapter, I explore the relationship between eugenics and genetics with these complexities in mind. I will begin by considering the history of eugenics and genetics from the early part of the twentieth century to the postwar era. I will refer back to the dichotomies in Box 2.1 in order to frame my analysis, but I will not deconstruct them systematically. Drawing on a range of historical and contemporary studies of eugenics and genetics, I will argue that eugenics cannot be consigned to the historical dustbin, but that its form has changed through time. I will argue that the genetics has both reflected and reinforced a variety of eugenic ideologies about the relationships between the individual, the state, disease and social order. However, I will not argue that the dichotomies of Box 2.1 can simply be collapsed, as critics of the new genetics would argue. Distinctions can still be drawn between certain aspects of eugenics and genetics. Although such distinctions are flexible and contingent upon the social circumstances in which they are drawn, they are not without analytical value.

I will go on to consider how the dichotomies of Box 2.1 are both invoked and rejected in contemporary discussions about eugenics and genetics, and on what grounds this occurs. To understand these processes, I will consider the social context of discussions about genetics and eugenics, especially the dynamics of expertise and governance. My focus is mainly British and American, but I remain mindful of the increasingly global character of genetics research and services and how this shapes the national context.

Surveillance, coercion and voluntarism

In this section, I will explore genetics and eugenics in the pre- and post Second World War periods, particularly the relationship between the eugenics movement and the emergent science of genetics, and ways in which eugenics has been associated with population policies based upon coercion and compulsion, on the one hand, and individuals' voluntary choices, on the other.

The beginning of the twentieth century was a time of considerable social turmoil in Britain. The urban poor were becoming a social problem, and the rise of militant labour was becoming a political problem. Concern mounted about the high fertility rates of the so-called underclasses, who it was thought passed on their propensity to feeble-mindedness and deviance to their off-spring. The state took on more responsibility for the welfare of its citizenry and the institutionalization of deviant and disabled people developed apace. A new middle class of professional doctors, warders and social reformers classified and supervised these underclasses. From their ranks, the leaders of the eugenics movement emerged. Eugenic ideas were popular with scientists, doctors, academics, educationalists, politicians and activists from a range of political positions, from feminism to conservatism. All shared an interest in preventing hereditary decline, and 'breeding' better Britons, primarily through limiting the birth of the lower classes and feeble-minded and encouraging the middle classes to procreate. These ideas soon became popular in the United States, where concerns about immigration meant eugenics was embedded in a racist ideology of white supremacy (Allen, 1983).

These beginnings of eugenics are intimately tied to the emerging sciences of genetics and psychology in particular. As Garland Allen has noted, a large number of serious and well-established biologists saw eugenics as a way of applying the principles of their discipline to the improvement of the population. The Lancet and the Royal College of Surgeons and Physicians made statements in support of eugenic sterilization. It was 'medical men' who were at the forefront of calls for so-called negative eugenics, with the aim of preventing degeneracy though restricting breeding and its practice: euthanasia of so-called 'defective children' and sterilization of the feeble-minded. Eugenics was taught in colleges and universities, without compunction. For example, a 1928 survey recording 343 out of 499 colleges in the USA offering courses in eugenics and genetics (Nelkin and Lindee, 1995).

There is no doubt that the values of eugenics also seeped into public health and child welfare policies in Britain. Mark Thomson (1998) shows the influence of eugenic thinking upon the institutionalization of disabled people, particularly the so-called feeble-minded. School inspections identified large numbers of ill and undernourished children, and generated yet more anxiety among professionals and government about the state of the British populace. The solution was public health measures such as improved sanitation, designed to improve the conditions of the masses and yet more institutionalization in workhouses, prisons and reformatories.

However, there was much pessimism about the ability of the masses to lift themselves out of poverty, a pessimism that was fuelled by the emergent science of genetics. The emphasis here was upon identifying hereditary rather than social reasons for inequalities. For example, Galton studied the inheritance of ability and IQ, and his results furthered the sense of pessimism about the prospects of the feeble-minded. Eugenics also shaped the emergent discipline of psychology, which had a strong emphasis upon surveillance – the Binet test, the forerunner to the IQ test. Sophisticated statistical techniques such as the Bell Curve owe their origins to eugenics. Many psychologists, school doctors and educators with eugenic sensibilities supported segregation of the mentally defective and voluntary sterilization, as did physicians from a range of medical specialisms. Eugenic sensibilities were particularly popular among professionals such as psychiatrists, who struggled to cure the increasing numbers of people diagnosed as mentally ill. It is therefore clearly not possible to dismiss these aspects of eugenics as mere pseudo-science, driven by ideologues rather than scientists.

Britain never took the more radical steps of eugenicists in other countries such as the United States where compulsory sterilization was widely practiced. Nor did the British State embark upon an overtly racist population policy, unlike the USA. Instead, the emphasis here was upon voluntarism, although that inevitably disguised the degree to which professionals undermined clients' autonomy in birth control practices. With reference to efforts to introduce a compulsory sterilization, Trombley notes in *The Right to Reproduce*,

> It had long been Havelock Ellis's view that the whole project of a sterilization bill was dangerous because it merely raised doubts in the minds of doctors who were sterilizing people anyway.
>
> (Trombley, 1988: 139)

These practices undermine the division between coercion and choice that is often made where eugenics and genetics are contrasted. This is not because genetics does not involve choice, as is sometimes argued, but because eugenics has also involved a discourse of choice, despite its reputation for overt coercion. Although I am not suggesting that these choices were entirely free (what choices ever are?), we cannot disregard this interest in voluntarism on the part of British eugenicists. A focus upon British and indeed American eugenics also undermines the association between eugenics and totalitarianism – eugenics clearly also flourished in liberal democracies.

The surveillance system in other countries, such as the United States, Sweden, and, of course, Germany, was on an altogether more sophisticated and brutal scale than the British arrangements. As US institutions became overcrowded, radical measures were favoured, and compulsory sterilization legislation passed in 30 states, with the support of many physicians and social reformers. In Germany, the Nazis' rise to power in dreadful economic and social conditions, meant that latent public and professional sympathy for involuntary euthanasia of defective children transformed into a widespread programme of genocide. We should also remember that German eugenicists were not entirely out of step with some of their American colleagues. Instead, they drew inspiration from the theories and practices of American eugenics, particularly compulsory sterilization. A widespread system of surveillance supported these barbaric practices. Teachers, doctors, other professionals, and even sometimes parents, reported so-called defectives to the appropriate authorities so that they could be sterilized. A wide range of ordinary bureaucrats also made sure that euthanasia programmes operated efficiently. By the end of the Second World War, around a quarter of a million people had been killed. Eugenics was also popular in many other regions, such Latin American, Japan and Scandinavia. Some countries, or states within them, made sterilization of certain groups of people compulsory; others relied upon encouraging individuals within these groups to volunteer to be sterilized. Experts in science and medicine were prominent supporters of these measures, seeing them as one route towards scientific and social progress in their respective countries.

It took several decades for some of the shine to wear off the ideology of supremacy that underlay these practices. The decline of what Kevles (1995) has called mainline eugenics is often attributed to widespread abhorrence of the excesses of the Nazi genocide. However, increasing debates within the scientific professions about the theories and evidence for eugenicists' claims, as well as opposition from the Catholic Church and the organized labour movement, also decreased the political viability of pathologizing the working classes in the postwar era.

Geneticists challenged eugenics in this period, and undermined its more flamboyant claims. However, they were slow to do so for fear of losing their institutional support and status. As Paul (1998) has argued, the consensus amongst geneticists about the role of heredity in determining behavioural as well as moral traits was also strong, and never at the root of their concerns. They may have been critical of the barbarism of eugenics, but they shared an interest in the improvement of the genetic constitution of the species. Genetics did lose status after the war, as scientists and clinicians stayed out of the limelight, working on a more modest scale in the laboratory and the clinic. The old values nevertheless remained, albeit in a more muted form. Genes were still thought to determine a range of diseases, traits and social problems. Directive counselling continued, so did sterilization without informed consent, and genetic studies of mental and behavioural disorders and traits, even when the term eugenics fell out of favour.

Latent eugenic sentiments about single parents and large working class families lingered. Francis Crick's and James Watson's discovery of the structure of DNA in 1953 gave Crick the opportunity to call, in 1961, for the establishment of a large-scale eugenics programme, which included the sterilization of the citizenry through food additives. As Diane Paul (1998) notes, throughout the 1960s most of the leading figures in medical genetics bluntly described their work as a form of eugenics.

Sterilization of poor and disabled women continued long after the war, on the grounds that they were unfit mothers. Up to 10,000 women were sterilized during abortions in UK between April 1968 and 1969. Right-wing British politicians such as Keith Joseph also continued to subscribe to notions of problem families and degeneracy well into the 1970s (Trombley, 1988). Mental defectives requiring permanent care were excluded from Beveridge's social citizenship and the introduction of universal benefits resulted in reduced provision for these groups who were viewed as a burden on the welfare state. More emphasis was placed upon voluntary treatment for less severe forms of mental illness in the British Mental Health Act (1959). Social controls that were previously achieved through institutionalization were now largely articulated through medicalization.

The contours of welfare provision and notions of social, political and economic citizenship in contemporary Britain have clearly changed since the postwar period. However, the so-called underclass and others deemed misfits by virtue of disability, anti-social behaviour or illness remain under the obligation to reform and conform in societies' interests. As we shall see in the section that follows, the language of obligation has shifted to a powerful discourse of individualism, but it is the broad link between past and present interests in the control of these groups that I wish to emphasize here.

Of course, these attitudes to anti-social behaviour, mental illness and disabilities, are no longer the key drivers of genetic research, as they were for some geneticists in the past. However, they do form the backdrop to an increasing interest in behavioural genetics, particularly around cognitive ability and attention deficit disorders. Distancing themselves from what they characterize as the abuses and bad science of the past, some behavioural geneticists claim to have amassed a huge amount of reliable data about the genetic basis of behaviours based on animal studies and twin and adoption studies

(Mann, 1994). It is also argued that the identification of behaviourally relevant genes, such as those involved in cognitive ability, will give greater insight into the environmental basis of differences in human behaviour (McGue and Bouchard, 1998). As Rose (2000) has suggested, these technologies could bring self-surveillance to these 'hard to reach groups', offering a route into the social whole, just as self-administered anti-psychotic drugs could offer psychiatric patients a place in the community. However, these technologies of surveillance are not yet widely available, which means that people with mental health problems are more likely to experience social exclusion of the traditional sort. It is only certain privileged groups who are now given the dubious privilege of governing their own selves (although the extent of their autonomy remains more apparent than real). Others with less material and physical resources continue to be subject to inspection and incarceration in their own homes or other controlled environments run by state and medical authorities. Recalcitrance has long been met with professional and bureaucratic antagonism. In this era of liberal capitalism, the boundary between social inclusion and exclusion is all too easily traversed by poor and disabled people.

Clearly, eugenics should not be boxed off into the pre-war era. The relationship between genetics and eugenics took various forms before and after 1945. Some scientists and doctors who studied genetics drew inspiration from eugenics, others focused upon denouncing it. Doctors both enacted and rejected eugenic measures in their encounters with patients. Eugenic policies with the aim of population improvement involved coercive measures to sterilize or murder certain groups considered to be defective. However, eugenicists have also recognized the importance of individuals' voluntary choices to avoid genetic disease throughout its history. Scientists' and doctors' interests in deviancy and disease also overlaps. The distinctions between eugenics and genetics outlined in Box 2.1 do not capture the diversity and range of these associations and practices, but they cannot be dismissed in their entirety.

Prevention

Negative eugenics is all about the prevention of degeneracy through various interventions in reproduction. The tools of prevention and the ideology of degeneracy that guided them, clearly evolved during the twentieth century. Notions of disease and disability hardened into medical categories, although this did not mean their social origins could be erased. The focus upon prevention also shifted into the antenatal clinic, as new technologies such as ultrasound scanning and amniocentesis developed and obsession with the feeble-minded diminished. We should not forget that the focus upon prevention was not unique to the postwar period: even when technologies such as amniocentesis did not exist, doctors counselled families about their risks of having a child with a genetic disorder and advised abstention from sex in high-risk cases. However, there is no doubt that the arrival of amniocentesis and the liberalization of abortion spurred the development of tests for chromosomal abnormalities, under the prevailing logic of prevention of disability. Genetic counselling focused upon explaining these procedures to clients, with the understanding that with the right information and advice they would take the rational course of action. As Paul notes, Sheldon Reed, who coined the phrase 'genetic counselling' in 1947, emphasized a non-directive, individual-centred approach, within a wider eugenic ideology where he sought to transmit the traits of the most intelligent. This notion of rationality was intimately tied to the development of genetic counselling in the years that followed. Kevles, for example, quotes Lionel Penrose as saying in 1969,

> [If patients behaved in a way] that would be considered generally to be reasonable... the results of skillful counselling, over a long period of years, will undoubtedly be to diminish, very slightly but progressively, the amount of severe hereditary disease in the population.
>
> (Kevles, 1995: 258)

This suggests that we cannot easily divide population concerns from concerns about the individual, as the two are clearly entwined. However, it would also be wrong to exaggerate the impact of these tests upon the population at large, or to over-emphasize the extent to which they were imposed by a paternalistic profession. Prenatal diagnosis only became available for a limited number of conditions in the 1970s and 1980s, one of which was cystic fibrosis (CF). By this time, the focus of genetic counselling was upon parental choice, and screening was justified as a response to parental demand, as the following quote illustrates:

> We have already referred to the express wish of parents for a reliable test that would allow them to have children without the risk of CF. This implies acceptance of abortion if the foetus is found to be affected, and is of course a personal decision.
>
> (Dodge and Ryley, 1982: 778)

The emphasis upon clients' responsibilities to prevent genetic disease shifted to their rights to access and act upon this type of genetic information, in the interests of reducing the risk of genetic disease. Counselling literature stressed the importance of dialogue and communication between patients and counsellors, in order that they might reach decisions wisely rather than reach wise decisions (Shiloh, 1996).

This did not mean that the importance of producing a normal child, or reducing the emotional and financial burden of disability, went unacknowledged. For example, Chapple states the public health perspective:

> Every expectant parent fears that their child will be born with some serious physical or mental disability. An even greater worry is that a disability

could be passed on in part or wholly from one generation of the family to the next because of a faulty gene. This may burden the parents not only with a lifetime of care for a handicapped child but also with unwarranted feelings of responsibility that they have caused their child to be damaged.

(Chapple, 1992: 579)

Others, particularly obstetricians, have also been positive about the benefits of these new technologies in terms of disease reduction. The literature on genetic screening often evaluates new techniques in terms of cost benefit arguments: for example comparing the cost of a Down's syndrome screening programme per Down's pregnancy terminated, with the cost of the lifetime care of someone with Down's syndrome (Wald *et al.*, 1998). This kind of screening is advocated because it benefits society, not just individuals. Today's hype about genetics as a route to personalized lifestyle planning belies the reality that the majority of genetic interventions take place antenatally. As I shall discuss in the next chapter, the discourse of individual choice also masks the many pressures on pregnant women to comply with testing, screening and termination: pressures that, although now applied more subtly, reflect traditional attitudes to disability and parental responsibility.

Preventative measures aimed at reducing genetic disorder and disease changed in the course of the twentieth century. However, this has not simply been a matter of the focus shifting from populations to individuals, coercion to choice, or deviance to disease. In practice, boundaries between all of these categories are blurred. Similarly, the development of genetics has not involved a simple shift away from a crude form of genetic reductionism; or, for that matter, a return to its reactionary ideals, as I will discuss in the next section.

Reductionism

Supporters of the new genetics often claim that the crude reductionism of eugenics has been superseded by sophisticated modern techniques of molecular biology. Geneticists do not privilege nature over nurture as was once the case, but treat the gene–environment interaction seriously. As Aravida Chakravarti and Peter Little have argued,

> If the past 50 years has seen the revolution of DNA, then the revolution cannot be completed without an appreciation of both genetic and environmental individuality; only then will individuals understand the meaning of their inheritance.

(Chakravati and Little, 2003: 412)

For opponents of the new genetics, it is much more clearly associated with reductionism, or, in a more convoluted phrase, geneticization, which means, broadly, that genetic factors become the principal explanation for an ever widening list of health problems and social conditions. Reductionism of this sort is often associated with eugenics. When proponents of the new genetics talk of the book of life or the code of codes (as provided by the HGP) they are accused of reductionist, eugenic thinking. Geneticization and genetic reductionism are also associated with reactionary political agendas, where the maintenance of the status quo is at stake, and the fixity of nature is invoked to justify it. Nelkin and Lindee have argued that what they call 'genetic essentialism' can serve these types of social agenda:

> Genetic explanations of behavior and disease appear to locate social problems within the ideology of individualism. ... And genetic explanations appear to provide a rational, neutral justification of existing social categories. ... The status of the gene – as a deterministic agent, a blueprint, a basis for social relations, and a source of good and evil – promises a reassuring certainty, order, predictability, and control.
>
> (Nelkin and Lindee, 1995: 196)

For example, genetic explanations for crime locate the cause of criminality in the genes and suggest that for criminality to be eliminated measures must be taken to eliminate the genes or their effects, either through reproductive interventions, as in the past, or by some kind of therapeutic intervention. In the case of potentially violent or anti-social individuals, there have been calls for preventative detention, electronic tagging or other surveillance. The new data emerging from behavioural genetics could be put to similar uses. As Rose argues,

> Biological criminology, here, is but one element in the more general rise of public health strategies of crime control, focusing on the identification of, and preventative intervention upon, aggressive, risky or monstrous anti-citizens.
>
> (Rose, 2000: 24)

Biological explanations for criminality could also be used to suggest that certain families have a propensity to criminality, and should therefore be subject to surveillance and preventative therapy. Critics argue that this takes attention away from the social conditions which give rise to criminal behaviours, particularly inequalities in people's access to resources. This is linked to eugenics in the sense that the 'germplasm' of the early eugenic literature was also associated with reductionist thinking – as it was 'a source of identity' which attests to the 'bodily origins of social problems' (Nelkin and Lindee, 1995: 36).

However, we must be wary of the reductionism within the story of genetic reductionism in its own right. As a rhetorical device, genetic reductionism is a crude descriptor of genetic theories and research in the past the present. As Howard Kaye (1997) has argued, it is wrong to equate the biological arguments of the eugenics era with conservative politics. Many of the people who adopted a neo-Darwinian philosophy that emphasized the laws of nature were, in fact, revolutionaries who wished to overturn the old order in favour of social improvement based upon humanitarian social selection. Although the discoveries of Weismann, Mendel and De Vries were seen by eugenicists as a boost to their campaign, genetics also undercut eugenics in the interwar years as evolution came to be seen as acting upon gene frequencies rather than individual organisms. By the 1960s, many scientists had rejected the idea that biology could be a guide to social policy.

Reductionism was, however, to take on an altogether more powerful form. The elucidation of the structure of DNA in 1953, alongside other discoveries by Murenberg and Mattaei and Monod, were interpreted in support of the fundamental unity of life. As Kaye argues, 'the philosophical spokesmen for molecular biology' promoted an 'aggressive, simplifying reductionist approach and attitude rather than a specific subject matter' (1997: 55) – a research strategy and a worldview. Tauber and Sarkar concur:

> Reductionism in molecular biology constitutes a research program that attempts to explain and understand biological systems completely in terms of the physical interactions of their parts.
>
> (Tauber and Sarkar, 1992: 228)

As Van Dijck notes, the Human Genome Project, the multi-billion dollar project to map the entire human genome, involved a new set of imagery that contrasts with the 'gene as controller' metaphors of the previous decades. Computing and informational metaphors strongly influenced the new notion of 'genome': a digital inscription of the genetic make-up (Van Dijck, 1998: 120). She continues,

> Invention and stimulation of methods like reverse genetics tacitly change the primary goal of the mapping project from defining the ideal (healthy) human being into defining its diseases or flaws. These goals might seem like two sides of the same coin, yet a strong emphasis on determining aberrations in the genetic make-up yields a view of the body as the flawed version of the perfect code, and concurrently holds the promise of an easy genetic fix.
>
> (Van Dijck, 1998: 122)

Clearly, molecular biology is associated with a much more powerful and all-encompassing form of genetic reductionism than the genetics of the past; but it is shaped by institutional and commercial interests in profit, more than it is by reactionary political agendas. Just as eugenics in the past spanned the political divide between left and right, a range of professionals and publics subscribe to some forms of genetic reductionism, and this cannot be explained by their political principles alone.

Some have argued that genetic reductionism will be undone by the discoveries of the HGP and the study of genetic disease. Around the time of the announcement of the draft human genome it was widely claimed that the identification of fewer than expected genes in the human genome (30,000 rather than 100,000) signalled 'the end of genetic determinism'. Evelyn Fox Keller has argued that,

> ... these very advances will necessitate the introduction of other concepts, other terms, and other ways of thinking about biological organization, thereby inevitably loosening the grip that genes have had on the imagination of the life scientists these many decades.
>
> (Keller, 2000: 147)

There is no doubt that many geneticists are acutely aware of genetic complexity. For example, more than one thousand mutations have been identified in cystic fibrosis, and it has proved very difficult to match the CF genotype with the phenotype (limiting scientists' ability to identify genes which result in mild or serious symptoms). However, genetic reductionism has not simply been overtaken by today's multi-gene paradigm. Identifying multiple genes involved in a group of disorders can still involve reductionism, depending upon how this knowledge is interpreted and applied. The complexities of the CF gene have not stalled the introduction of antenatal CF screening in the United States. This screening is the product of public health goals of reducing the incidence of genetic disease, alongside the political need for large-scale government initiatives such as the HGP to demonstrate their usefulness. These programmes also create a jurisdictional foothold over the implementation of new genetic technologies for groups like obstetricians. These types of political and professional drivers can undercut more holistic analyses of genes and their biological and social environments now, as in the past.

So far, I have questioned any stark divide between past eugenics and present-day genetics on the basis of the types of knowledge or forms of social controls that they have involved. Eugenics can be 'pinned down' to a simple set of values or practices, such as population improvement or state-sanctioned coercion. Eugenics has also been associated with an ideology of voluntarism and choice. However, genetic reductionism and social control through surveillance and prevention have changed in the course of the last two hundred years. The individual is privileged more than ever before, as are the complexities of genes. Yet the pathologization of certain forms of 'deviant' behaviour and the focus upon medical rather than social solutions to disability and disease remain.

Why, then, do the dichotomies of Box 2.1 continue to have such force? The answer to this question is not as simple as it might first appear. In other words, these dichotomies are not simply the product of professional humbug. They are adopted by a range of different groups, to support a range of different practices. Sometimes they are 'debunked' in arguments against one technology, but are deployed in arguments in support of another. They are clearly flexible boundaries, rather than absolutes. It is this flexibility that means they endure. Flexible discourses suit the contemporary era, given that people's relationships, identity and status are multiple and fluid. The complex interlocking of commerce, government and expertise make lines of demarcation between these domains and the people within them far from clear. I now turn to explore the ways in which this wider context relates to a range of different discourses about eugenics where the dichotomies of Box 2.1 are flexibly deployed.

Commerce, governance and expertise

Commercial interest in genetics grew rapidly in the 1970s. In the United States, the state was key to the development of the biotechnology industry in the 1970s and 1980s, actively encouraging commercial investment and growth (Wright, 1986). As corporate biotechnology expanded, the always artificial divide between knowledge and technique, or science and technology, eroded, and patent applications mushroomed. Small-scale biotechnology companies were swallowed, or controlled via shareholdings and contracts, by multinational firms. Trading in patents meant sale to the highest bidder. Patent ownership became concentrated in the hands of a few pharmaceutical giants, who had the capacity to enforce the patent in the way that small-scale organizations cannot. These corporations also had considerable lobbying power, and were able to achieve significant regulatory changes in the United States during the Reagan era, where as Susan Wright notes, the emphasis shifted from 'protection against the effects of technology to protection for its rapid development' (Wright, 1986: 337). For example, the Patent and Trademark Amendment Act of 1980 gave 'universities, small businesses, and non-profit organizations rights to patents arising from federally supported research' (ibid.: 338). As a consequence, Wright notes, 'commercial norms with respect to scientific practice replaced academic norms, and commercial goals penetrated deep into the design of research' (ibid.: 360).

This has directly involved many geneticists in share ownership and patent applications as the university and commercial sector focused upon protecting their investments in the potentially lucrative area of genetics-based health screening and treatments. A range of organizations such as Cancer Research UK and the Human Genome Organization (HUGO) are just as focused upon negotiating ownership of and access to genetic information as they are upon facilitating basic research into the genetic aspects of disease. Public–private partnership is now key, as the following quote from the HGP information website illustrates:

> An important feature of this project is the federal government's long-standing dedication to the transfer of technology to the private sector. By licensing technologies to private companies and awarding grants for innovative research, the project is catalyzing the multibillion-dollar U.S. biotechnology industry and fostering the development of new medical applications.
> (http://www.ornl.gov/hgmis/home.html)

At the turn of the century, there were many thousands of patents on human DNA. The 35,000–40,000 genes identified in the working draft of the genome, although well short of the 100,000 initially predicted, is nevertheless a large number of genes with significant commercial potential. Gene patenting is also likely to thrive, as the regulatory context is lax, as Bobrow and Thomas comment:

> In the absence of serious legislative action, policy has more or less evolved through dialogue within a limited circle of participants. Commercial interests, which are well represented to the patent offices, have not been counter-balanced by those who represent the broader public interest. The result has been an innate tendency for the patent system to 'creep' in the direction of extending patentability to biotechnology inventions for which the thresholds for novelty, inventiveness and utility have been lowered.
>
> (Bobrow and Thomas, 2001: 763–4)

However, commercial interests in genetics are controversial, particularly where patenting or secrecy might stifle the innovation of new tests and treatments (see Sulston and Ferry, 2002).

As Webster and Nelis (1999) have argued, regulation is now highly flexible, and open to perpetual negotiation. It is not possible to identify a clear and dominant standpoint amongst the plethora of policy-making bodies about what should be regulated, let alone how it should be regulated. Multiple strategies for control mirror stakeholders' multiple interests. Much of what currently passes for regulation therefore involves non-statutory guidelines or recommendations. Continuous monitoring has taken the place of top-down enforcement. Policies are necessarily flexible to reflect the fluid and transitory relationships from which they develop and evolve. Even when regulatory mechanisms coalesce in the form of practice guidelines, for example, their articulation in practice is far from predictable or uniform. Instead, a range of informal local practices and moral codes mediate their implementation.

However, this flexibility does not suggest a regulatory free-for-all. The actors with an interest in genetic policy-making do not have the same amount of influence over its eventual outcome. The market place is particularly influential in shaping the contemporary governance of science and medicine. Public and private collaborations fund biomedical research, as well as hospital building programmes and academic institutions. Consumer sovereignty has become a key value in relation to public as well as private services. Not only do the priorities of the private sector directly impinge upon policy-making and service provision where they are directly involved, but the associated value of consumer choice implicitly shapes the public sector.

This is not to say that the market has simply been left to its own devices. Rather, the market and the state negotiate governance, in an effort to maximize their individual and mutual benefits. The state has assumed a certain mantle of responsibility for protecting consumers from the vagaries of the market. As such, the state must also be seen to be a responsible, discriminating, consumer in its own right, hence the appeal of evidence-based medicine, best practice and auditing practices such as benchmarking. The allied logic of balancing citizens' rights and responsibilities has also meant that the state has devolved a certain amount of governance to individuals, who must now assume responsibility for their own health.

Contemporary debates about eugenics

Genetic research and services are a part of this calculus of national competitiveness, devolved governance, and localized practices. The flexible, de-centred approach of contemporary governance is said by some to foster a form of *laissez-faire*, individualized eugenics. However, others claim that pluralized liberal democracy is the best way to undermine eugenics. The discourses of eugenics are therefore both topics and resources for contemporary governance. Beck (1993) puts another twist on this when he argues that the widely perceived inadequacies of expert-led governance have resulted in new forms of institutional reflexivity and sub-politics that revitalize participatory democracy. This suggests that the public can choose to reject what they see as new forms of individualized, commercialized eugenics.

Modern nation states and their international conglomerates tend to favour professional self-regulation through non-statutory advisory bodies, and emphasize individual choice of patients and consumers. UNESCO's Universal Declaration on the Human Genome and Human Rights (adopted on 11 November 1997) was among the first international guidelines to be produced on the human genome. Reflecting the current emphasis upon the individual, the declaration emphasized their right to respect their dignity and rejected genetic determinism. It seeks a balance between ethical concerns and scientific progress, supporting genetic services for serious diseases with proper counselling services, but rejects reproductive cloning because of its eugenic overtones. This liberal approach is seen as an important bulwark against latent eugenic impulses that might be harboured by nation states and their bureaucrats. The *WHO Proposed International Guidelines on Ethical Issues in Medical Genetics and Genetic Services* (1998) take a similar stance, favouring genetic services based around the principles of informed choice, confidentiality, equity of access, and public education about genetics. It is often argued that the benefits of gene technologies in terms of economic prosperity and the alleviation of suffering outweigh its potential disadvantages. Restrictive legislation is resisted on the basis that allowing scientists to pursue this research and parents to decide on how to use any information that is generated, mediates against eugenics, because eugenics is a matter of governmental policy, not individual choice (Gordon, 1999).

In countries such as Germany, this liberal approach is, however, controversial, given the Nazi legacy. Genetic research on embryos is strongly resisted by many sections of German society because it instrumentalizes life and could be used to enable ambitious parents to differentiate between worthy and unworthy embryos, fuelling a commercial form of eugenics. The eugenic implications of embryo research and genetic enhancement are especially contested. The strength of the anti-abortion movement in the United States also means that this is an import issue there too. However, not all of the criticisms of these developments concern the sanctity of the embryo. As Jeremy Rifkin has argued,

> We are on the cusp of a commercial Eugenics Era. . . . The question of whether commercial enterprises would be allowed to own human beings as property before birth will likely be one of the seminal political issues of the Biotech Century. . . . Failure to examine the commercial implications of embryo and stem cell research could trap us in a commercial eugenics future that we neither anticipated or chose.
>
> (Rifkin, 2001)

Here Rifkin draws parallels between state-control and commercial-control, in this case, over the ownership of life. For critics like Rifkin, embryo and stem cell research and technologies for selecting and/or improving embryos or foetuses are supply-driven rather than demand-led. The capitalist drive for profit is akin to the state drive for perfection. Consumer choice is a mere illusion. Other critics have labelled these technologies 'yuppie eugenics' on the grounds that choice is a myth and the underlying goal of improvement of the species remains.

> A contemporary, ostensibly voluntary form of older ideas and practices, Yuppie Eugenics is based in modern molecular genetics and concepts of 'choice', and has begun to raise the high tech prospect of employing prenatal genetic engineering. What it shares with the earlier doctrines is the goal of improving and perfecting human bloodlines and the human species as a whole.
>
> (Hubbard and Newman, 2002)

For others, these choices are real. These technologies are a benign form of eugenics, given that they are designed with the aim of giving couples more choices about their future progeny, and that the desire for the perfect child is both widespread and utterly reasonable. As *The Economist* puts it,

> The case for most sorts of human cloning is simple and similar to IVF: it will allow people who cannot reproduce to do so. . . . Parents can already select which particular embryo to implant, so as to screen out specific diseases. In the long run, modifying these embryos offers a chance to practise a benign form of eugenics: for parents to eliminate undesirable traits from their children. So long as these traits are medical conditions, this seems acceptable.
>
> (Anonymous, 2001)

The history of compulsory sterilization and the politics of abortion, alongside the general unwillingness of states to restrict emergent health care markets, have resulted in a profound emphasis upon couples' right to choose the characteristics of their future children. Already highly medicalized and costly, both emotionally and financially, assisted reproduction is not in the business of producing imperfect children. Why implant a less than perfect embryo when you can choose to avoid this?

For some, especially bioethicists, this means that couples electing not to implant genetically weak embryos are not engaged in anything akin to the eugenics of the past. For example, John Harris has argued that the use of these technologies on an individual basis extends choice to people who might otherwise not have children. As long as this technology is available to all, without compulsion, he claims it does not constitute immoral eugenics. For Harris, eugenics is immoral when a majority of people force a certain minority to use these technologies of selective breeding (Harris, 1993). As Reindal has argued, this argument rests on an individualized, biological explanation of disability and treats the users of these technologies as individual consumers, rather than members of particular social groups (Reindal, 2000).

Other bioethicists, such as Julian Savulescu, share this *laissez-faire* approach to new genetic technologies, arguing that people must be allowed to act on their own conception of the good life in liberal democracy, even if this involves them in what might be considered non-medical choices, about the sex of their progeny, for example (Savulescu, 2001). As Savulescu continues, what he calls procreative beneficence is different to eugenics:

> Eugenics is selective breeding to produce a better population. A public interest justification for interfering in reproduction is different from Procreative Beneficence which aims at producing the best child of the possible children. That is an essentially private enterprise.
>
> (Savulescu, 2001: 424)

Similar arguments are also made with respect to lifting restrictions of germline genetic engineering. Engelhardt has argued, for example,

> In a postmodern world, humans face the challenge of directly shaping their own evolution, although they share no common understanding of human destiny and purpose.
>
> (Engelhardt, 2002: 169)

Policy-making bodies and professionals nevertheless tend to draw the line at the use of these technologies to select embryos on so-called non-medical grounds, because this would deny the resultant child dignity and autonomy (Anonymous, 2001). Regulatory bodies such as the UK Human Fertilization and Embryology Authority (HFEA) and many of the health professionals working in assisted conception, also seek to draw clear distinctions between preimplantation diagnosis to avoid serious genetic disorders and non-medical selection, on the basis that the latter is a step too far in the direction of eugenics. Similar lines are drawn between somatic and germ-line gene therapy or between enhancement and prevention of disease – passing on improvements to future generations is classed as eugenic.

Professional groups associated with genetics use the dichotomies of Box 2.1 in a range of ways. They tend to reject the polarized visions of the trailblazers and the critics of the new eugenics, as discussed earlier, and to draw their own lines between acceptable forms of commercial links in genetics. They are ambivalent about the availability of genetic information to insurance companies because of fears of discrimination, but they are ambivalent about gene patenting because it could limit access to testing. Although they want genetic services to expand, if this were to take place without the widespread availability of professional counselling, they have expressed concerns about the danger of eugenics (Kerr *et al.*, 1998a; Cunningham-Burley and Kerr, 1999; Billings, 2000). They also argue that many of the claims about future genetic enhancements are fanciful in the extreme (Ewbank, 1998). On the other hand, they reject the accusation that they are working towards eradicating disabled people, and emphasize the important of non-directive counselling and individual choice, as we have already seen.

Yet divisions between these professional groups inevitably remain, both nationally and internationally. Mention of eugenics is one way of establishing and maintaining these boundaries. For example, we can find parallels between the way in which UK scientists used accusations of eugenics to degrade their US counterparts in debates around Mendelianism at the beginning of the twentieth century, and current discussions about the eugenic potential of national DNA databases such as the Icelandic database (see Chapter 6). The recent British white paper (Department of Health 2003a) about the future of genetics performs similar national 'boundary work' when it sets the future of genetics within the context of the NHS, which is described as providing a 'bulwark against the inequalities and inefficiencies of private insurance', in contrast with the USA (see Chapter 8). Suggestions of eugenics, explicitly or implicitly, continue to be used by scientists and technocrats when advocating new developments in which they would play a central part.

Other divisions also exist within the genetics field, for example between clinical and molecular genetics, or between medical and behavioural genetics, as the following quote from a discussion with a clinical geneticist about behavioural genetics illustrates:

> I find it all very iffy and I wouldn't touch it with a barge pole personally. It hasn't impinged on my practice at all so it's just my views [based] on reading it like anyone else. I don't find the gay gene convincing. I don't think the base is good enough. And I think a lot of the schizophrenia stuff that's come out, a lot of that is very iffy . . . at the end of the day I'm sure there is a pure genetic schizophrenia. But, it's like cancer genetics, it's a predisposition and it's not all or nothing. And once you get onto these multifactorial [conditions] I think genetics becomes less useful.

And that's why I'm sceptical of this genetic fingerprint of us all ... And that gets away from my job actually. I think when a gene gives you a twenty percent chance of something ... of a common thing ... it's actually not terribly useful information in the end.

(Kerr *et al.*, 1998a)

The 'iffiness' in part stems from a sense that the knowledge-base of behavioural genetics is suspect, but it is also related to its eugenic overtones (see also Cunningham-Burley and Kerr, 1999).

Non-professionals can also become involved in these discussions. Rabinow (1996) emphasizes the importance of new forms of biomedical subjectivity, and the important role in which patients now play in finding out about their condition. This goes beyond an individual search for knowledge, as support groups are formed by people with the condition, the project becomes one of building communities, and sometimes also challenging medical authority.

We must be careful not to exaggerate the extent to which these groups represent an antidote to professional expertise, or, indeed, eugenic thinking. People do not necessarily participate in the organizations that are supposed to represent their interests and many place a premium upon acquiring and spreading orthodox forms of expertise. However, there are clearly more of these types of patient-led organizations in the contemporary age. They participate in discussions about eugenics, alongside experts, drawing boundaries between past and present to support their particular cause. For example, The UK Genetics Interest Group (GIG), an umbrella organization representing genetic support groups, has produced a document where they argue that,

In GIG's view, both the ethos and the science of medical genetics are quite different from historical eugenics. Medical genetics is neither 'reductionist' nor morally discriminatory. Rather, the underlying spirit of the field is to consider people equal as human beings, while recognising that some have, or are at risk of producing children with, a medical condition. Clearly, selective implantation and termination are not 'cures'. However, the spirit of the new genetics is a search for the alleviation of disease and suffering, which often takes the path of pre-implantation diagnosis or selective termination of pregnancy precisely because cures are not available. The attitudes of parents and, in large part society as a whole, to fetal abnormality reflect attitudes towards illness – they feel sympathy for the ill and they want to cure them. They do not want to marginalise still less eradicate them.

(Genetic Interest Group, 1999)

Experts in genetics and people affected by genetic disease also come together to challenge what they view as discriminatory behaviour on the part of other agencies, such as insurance companies, and in so doing defend the boundaries between genetics and eugenics. Genetics professionals clearly have an interest in people making use of the services they offer, and the widespread availability of their results to a range of third parties might make people less willing to be tested. Concerns about stigma and discrimination by non-experts are given as reasons to keep this knowledge confidential. Such stigma has echoes of the discrimination involved in the eugenics of the past, and its basis in what is cast as misuse of the science. It is therefore sometimes in experts' and disabled people's interests to invoke the spectre of eugenics in their campaigns to limit access to genetic information. For example, investigative journalist Edwin Black has written,

> ...'newgenics' has risen to again persecute and discriminate on the basis of blood ancestry. Insurance companies, employers and others want to exclude those deemed to be insurance risks and even socially unacceptable.
>
> (Black, 2003)

(See also The International Sub-Committee of BCODP statement on The New Genetics and Disabled People, 2000, http://www.bcodp.org.uk/about/genetics.html and Holtzman and Rothstein, 1992.)

Although a considerable proportion of these discussions concern future technologies, that are not yet available, they are an important part of the discussions about the links or otherwise between genetics and eugenics. For many bioethicists, the location of these technologies in consumer markets means that they are different from eugenics, where the state sought to improve the population by limiting the kinds of people who could breed. Couples will soon be able to choose to have children, whereas in the past they would have remained childless. They will be able to decide for themselves the kinds of children they want to have, just as they will decide to what extent they will modify their own health and lifestyles in response to genetic risk. Their opinions on what counts as acceptable and unacceptable deficiencies will vary. Benign, new or moral eugenics, are based upon a social model where the individual is all-powerful.

For critics from the ecological, feminist and disability movements, consumption will be the vehicle for, not the solution to, eugenics. The quest for perfection remains the underlying goal of the people who will develop, implement and use these technologies. Large organizations, be they the state or commerce, will seek control of the means by which people select the lives of their future progeny, patenting genes and standardizing screening programmes: encouraging the quest for perfection. Although they view these developments with horror, they share their opponents' sense of people's appetite for choice, and of scientists' and clinicians' ability to offer such choices. For both sides in the debates, genetic technologies are transformative.

Both of these groups are keen to stake their ground in the decentred and flexible regulatory regimes concerned with these new genetic developments. However, their pronouncements often fail to capture the ambivalence about the commercialization of genetics and its associations with eugenics as expressed by groups with a more direct stake in these developments, including, consumers, patients, corporations, professionals and regulators. Their views on consumer choice and technological capacity are often more circumspect. Experts have repositioned themselves as more reflexive and less didactic actors in the policy-making arena. A range of different notions of eugenics are mobilized in these discussions. Eugenics can be a form of coercion, but it can also be the abuse of neutral scientific information. Health professionals often disassociate genetic tests from eugenics on the basis of individual choice over the management of disease; but they caution that if these tests were to be offered without adequate counselling and the results became widely available, eugenic discrimination might occur. Alliances between experts and other stakeholders are also flexible as they variously defend certain practices against accusations of eugenics, at the same time as they raise concerns about eugenics in other areas of contemporary practice. For example, clinical geneticists might support preimplantation genetic diagnosis at the same time as they reject developments in behavioural genetics because of their eugenic potential. At times, disabled people and patients will be their allies, for example in restricting commercial access to genetic information, at other times they may come into conflict over their focus upon prenatal testing rather than support services, for example. Although eugenics has always had these varied meanings, and experts have always disagreed about its scientific basis and its social worth, it is probably fair to say that today's discussions are particularly marked by contingency and ambivalence as reflexivity and shifting alliances become more visible, and perhaps more socially acceptable. Just as expertise is flexible, so too are conceptions of eugenics.

Conclusion

> The melancholy refrain of those who...convict all references to the biological of reductionism, individualism and determinism, or who predict a new eugenics, are of little help in understanding the issues at stake [in the politics of life].
>
> (Rose, 2001: 22)

As Nikolas Rose argues, it is important to be wary of blanket condemnation of the new genetics on the basis of its eugenics associations. It is clear that because 'eugenics' has never had one fixed meaning, across different social groups, or different times, any rigid divisions or associations between scientific practices and ideologies are artificial constructs. Instead, we must accept that both history and the present are disordered, and explore the contradictory and the anomalous in both science and society.

When thinking about eugenics and genetics, it is important to be mindful of the different meanings and practices of each, and how this is located in particular cultural and historical contexts. It is also important to unpack the strong rhetorical function of appeals to genetics or appeals to/accusations of eugenics. In noticing some of the common threads that run through these different historical periods, particularly the emphasis on prevention of genetic disabilities and diseases, we should also stress the disparate trends in both ideology and practice. This means that whilst we must not fall into the trap of only seeing strong and enduring parallels between the past and the present, as highlighted by Rose, we must also be wary of exaggerating the differences between the past and the present.

The dichotomies of Box 2.1 can be found in contemporary discussions about the implications of commercialism in genetics, the best forms of genetic governance, and the lines between acceptable and unacceptable practices. The ways in which they are deployed reflect the flexible relationships between consumers, companies, experts and policy-makers, who form various alliances in support or opposition to particular developments, be they technological or regulatory, and tailor their discourse of eugenics accordingly. For some commentators, commercial involvement in genetics, and devolved governance foster liberty; for others liberty can only be protected by restrictions on commercialization through strict legislation. Alliances and discourse shifts according to the genetic technologies or forms of genetic information in question. These are highly flexible discourses, reflecting the flexible relationships and identities of their authors. It would therefore be naive to assume that, as their roles in contemporary discussion about genetics are exposed, so they will atrophy. Instead, the spectre of eugenics, in all its guises, will undoubtedly remain, for critics and advocates of genetics alike.

Further reading

Kerr, A. and Shakespeare, T. (2002) *Genetic Politics: From Eugenics to Genome*, Cheltenham: New Clarion Press.

Kerr, A., Cunningham-Burley, S. and Amos, A. (1998a) 'Eugenics and the new genetics in Britain: examining contemporary professionals' accounts', *Science, Technology & Human Values*, 23:2, 175–98.

Paul, D. (1992) 'Eugenic anxieties, social realities and political choices', *Social Research*, 59:3, 663–83.

Paul, D. (1998) *Controlling Human Heredity: 1865 to the Present*, New York: Humanity Books.

Rose, N. (2001) 'The politics of life itself', *Theory, Culture and Society*, 18:6, 1–30.

3 Discovery

Summary

In this chapter, I consider the ways in which genetic discoveries tend to be represented in popular formats such as the institutional press release, and how this deletes the complex ways in which social and economic relations, as well as the physical material with which scientists work, produce 'discoveries'. I am especially interested in the commercial context of genetic research, and the processes of governance as discussed in Chapter 2, and how these conditions shape scientists' ways of finding out about the world and the very processes by which things get to be called 'discoveries'. I also spend time discussing the relationship between the physical and the social aspects of disease, and where genes fit, or do not fit, onto definitions and explanations of disease.

  I begin with a press release, which I then go on to deconstruct in the course of the chapter. I focus upon the different actors involved in the process of discovery – commercial, regulatory, patient, professional and material. In each section, I draw on a range of empirical studies of genetic research and its social context, and link the findings of these studies to the case discussed in the press release. I conclude by reflecting upon how these different actors and the relationships between them shape what counts as a genetic discovery.

Introduction

When we think of genetics we tend to think of genetic discoveries. As Van Dijck (1998) has noted, the image of the geneticist as a hero discovering new land, hunting for treasure, mapping or conquering new territory, is a powerful one. Biotechnology becomes an adventure story, a journey that will bring prosperity and glory. Genomic mappers become medical heroes, ferreting out nature's secrets. This is particularly true when it comes to popular media accounts of genetics, which often begin, 'Scientists have discovered the gene for...'. As Peter Conrad has argued, this version of genetic discovery is linked to a pervasive form of genetic determinism. He argues that popular news often perpetuates what he calls the illusion of specific aetiology, or the 'one gene one disease' (OGOD) thesis (Conrad, 1999). In another paper, Conrad and Weinberg (1996) ask, rhetorically, 'has the gene for alcoholism been discovered three times since 1980?' to underline the persistent skew towards these deterministic narratives. They point out that research findings which suggest a link between genetics and alcoholism are given much more attention than studies which often go on to disprove the original research. The news media appears to have no memory of these prior claims and counterclaims, little scepticism or caution about the scientific claims, and a voracious appetite for dramatic stories and easy answers to complex social problems. A second feature of contemporary accounts of the new genetics that Conrad points out is the privileging of the role of genes as if they were independent of their environment. News stories tend to focus on the internal environment of DNA, not its environmental context. So we see stories such as those about *BRCA1*, a gene linked to only 5 per cent of breast cancers, where the genetics takes centre stage and environmental factors are secondary considerations. Third, Conrad notes that genes are part of a mechanistic view of the human body. Faulty genes are depicted as the causes of disease or behaviour – fix the gene and solve the problem. Yet genes do not work like that, they are part of a wider biological environment, which shapes and is shaped by their expression.

We habitually think of science and medicine in this way: scientists identify natural elements and intervene to allow us to capitalize on this knowledge, either to cure defects or to develop technologies that 'improve on nature'. This discourse developed at the time of the scientific revolution, where, as Evelyn Fox Keller puts it, nature became 'deanimated, desanctified, and increasingly mechanized' (Keller, 1985: 45). As Carol Merchant has argued,

> A cultural research program extending from the seventeenth century to the present day has resulted in mechanical models of the self, society, and the cosmos... nature can be divided into parts and the parts can be rearranged to create other species of being, 'Facts' or information bits can be extracted from the environmental context and rearranged according to a set of rules based on logical and mathematical operations.
>
> (Merchant, 1980: 164)

Although the masculine metaphor is less obvious in contemporary accounts, the discourse of unveiling nature's secrets remains in some of the more populist accounts of scientific discovery, and is reflected in allusions to science as a form of enlightenment or as a way of mining the rich resources of the natural world.

I will begin this chapter by deconstructing a press release about genetic discovery to explore the ways in which genes, disease, professionals, patients and knowledge are represented therein. I move on to consider the social context of genetic research, particularly, commercialism, governance, and professional relationships, and how they come to be deleted in the discovery discourse. I also consider the ways in which genes and diseases are co-produced, in order to show that the processes of discovering a gene are highly complex.

For immediate release
Monday, April 28, 2003   Contact:
Geoff Spencer
(301) 402-0911

Gene discovery opens door to further research in inherited neurological disorders
Charcot-Marie-Tooth and distal spinal muscular atrophy gene may shed light on Carpel Tunnel Syndrome and Lou Gehrig's disease

Bethesda, Maryland – Scientists at the National Human Genome Research Institute (NHGRI) and at the National Institute of Neurological Disorders and Stroke (NINDS) have identified the gene responsible for two related, inherited neurological disorders, and have, for the first time, directly implicated this gene and its enzyme product in a human genetic disease.

The discovery supports further investigation of this gene family for additional neurological disease genes, research that may shed light on a range of disorders, including carpel tunnel syndrome, which affects the hands and the wrists, and the fatal degenerative disease amyotrophic lateral sclerosis (ALS), also known as Lou Gehrig's disease.

NHGRI and NINDS scientists, working together at the National Institutes of Health (NIH), found the gene responsible for Charcot-Marie-Tooth (CMT) disease type 2D and distal spinal muscular atrophy (dSMA) type V. The gene, called *GARS* – the glycyl tRNA synthetase gene – is located on chromosome 7 and encodes, or provides the instructions to make, one of the aminoacyl tRNA synthetases, a family of enzymes vital to the cell's ability to build proteins.

'The identification of the defective gene on chromosome 7 responsible for a type of Charcot-Marie-Tooth disease provides another vivid example of how the recently completed human genome sequence is accelerating studies in human genetics', said Francis S. Collins, MD, PhD, director of NHGRI. 'With this discovery, we now know that the *GARS* gene – whose function is so fundamental to biological processes – can be mutated in a fashion that results in a highly discrete neurological disease.'

The study, a collaboration between the laboratories of Eric Green, MD, PhD, at NHGRI, Kenneth Fischbeck, MD, at NINDS, and Lev Goldfarb, MD, also at NINDS, will be available online in April and published in the May issue of the *American Journal of Human*

Genetics. Lead author Anthony Antonellis, a graduate student in Dr Green's laboratory, directed the project.

The scientists identified four disease-related mutations and speculate that a mutated copy of *GARS* leads to a reduction in the activity of the gene's enzyme product. More research into why this disruption produces the specific symptoms of CMT type 2D and dSMA type V will be necessary.

'Identifying this chromosome 7 disease gene at this particular time was especially gratifying in light of the recent completion of a finished sequence of this chromosome', said Dr Green, who is the Scientific Director of NHGRI and chief of its Genome Technology Branch. Dr Green also directs the NIH Intramural Sequencing Center. His laboratory has been involved in mapping and sequencing chromosome 7 as part of the Human Genome Project.

'This discovery is another piece of a jigsaw puzzle picture of how peripheral nerve diseases and motor neuron diseases happen', said Dr Fischbeck, chief of the Neurogenetics Branch at NINDS. Dr Fischbeck's laboratory studies hereditary motor neuron diseases and peripheral neuropathies. 'It provides a more complete view of the mechanism of these diseases. This will hopefully lead to new treatment approaches. The more complete the picture, the more we know how to intervene.'

Charcot-Marie-Tooth disease, named after the three physicians who first reported it in 1886, is a group of genetic diseases that causes muscle weakness and wasting, or atrophy, in the feet, legs, hands and forearms, as well as diminished sensation in the limbs. CMT disease affects the peripheral nerves – the nerves that travel to the muscles of the limbs – and is therefore known as a peripheral neuropathy. Estimated to affect one in 2,500 individuals, it is the most common inherited neurological disorder.

Some forms of CMT disease are autosomal dominant, meaning that a person needs to inherit only one defective copy of the responsible gene to acquire the disease. Other forms are autosomal recessive, meaning both copies of the gene must be defective to result in illness. There is also a form of CMT that is X-linked, meaning that the responsible gene is located on the X chromosome, one of the two sex chromosomes.

In most cases, CMT disease begins with mild symptoms, typically foot and ankle weakness and fatigue. As atrophy progresses, the patient develops a distinct walk, a consequence of muscle weakness in the front of the leg: the feet slap with each step and the body may sway from side to side. Eventually the toes and the fingers curl due to weakness and atrophy in the small muscles of the feet and the hands. Writing and other functions of the hands become difficult. The sensory loss that accompanies the atrophy diminishes the patient's ability to distinguish between hot and cold and affects the patient's sense of touch.

Persons with CMT disease usually begin to experience symptoms in adolescence or early adulthood. There is no cure for the disease, but there are treatment options, including physical therapy and bracing. Life expectancy is usually normal. CMT disease can be divided into two classes, depending on where the dysfunction occurs in the peripheral nerves. In CMT type 1, the peripheral nerves' axons — the part of the nerve cell that transmits electrical signals to the muscles — lose their protective outer coverings, their myelin sheaths. This disrupts the axons' function. In CMT type 2, the axons' responses are diminished due to a defect within the axons themselves.

CMT type 2, the less common of the two classes, can be further separated into at least six subtypes, caused by defects in different genes. The *GARS* gene is implicated in CMT type 2D, a form of CMT that primarily affects the hands and the forearms. CMT type 2D is inherited in an autosomal dominant fashion.

Spinal muscular atrophy (SMA) refers to a group of genetic diseases more diverse than those of CMT. SMA is characterized by weakness and wasting of the muscles of the limbs, but the types vary greatly in severity. Most common are autosomal recessive childhood-onset forms that may be fatal. Other types of SMA are inherited in an autosomal dominant fashion. All types of SMA are due to the degeneration of nerve cells within the spinal cord, as opposed to degeneration of the peripheral nerves.

Distal spinal muscular atrophy disease is a type of SMA that affects the hands and the feet. The *GARS* gene is implicated in dSMA type V. Its symptoms of muscle weakness and atrophy in the hands and the forearms mirror those of CMT type 2D, except that people with dSMA type V do not experience sensory loss. dSMA type V is also an autosomal dominant genetic disorder, like CMT type 2D.

Even though the *GARS* gene is implicated in only two specific types of CMT and SMA, this discovery will guide researchers in studying other forms of these diseases, as well as other neurological disorders. Because carpel tunnel syndrome affects the hands and the forearms, scientists may now investigate whether the *GARS* gene plays some role in this disorder. And two defective forms of the gene implicated in Lou Gehrig's disease are known to interact with a *GARS* family member.

Ultimately, the *GARS* gene and its family may provide a rich new resource for scientists investigating inherited and non-inherited neurological diseases.

'The next step is to explore what it is about motor nerve cells that make them particularly vulnerable to mutations in these genes', said Dr Fischbeck.

NHGRI is one of the 27 institutes and centers at the National Institutes of Health, which is an agency of the Department of Health and Human Services. The NHGRI Division of Intramural Research develops and implements technology to understand, diagnose and treat genomic and genetic diseases. Additional information about NHGRI can be found at its web site http://www.genome.gov

The discovery discourse

Consider the press release in Box 3.1. Although more conservative than many of these types of accounts in the popular press, this press release does reflect the determinist and linear model of discovery discussed earlier. Phrases like 'the gene responsible for', 'fundamental function' and 'rich resource' suggest reductionism. At the same time, the focus upon 'accelerating' studies of human genetics, 'shedding light' on gene function, taking the 'next step', piecing together the 'jigsaw puzzle' and 'guiding' future research, suggest progress and enlightenment through knowledge. The emphasis upon intervention and resources also suggests a capitalist system of exchange: research for the purpose of widening the market, in this case, in treatment. CMT is described by objective medical criteria, and the function of the gene is foregrounded, even though it is not implicated in many types of the condition. Scientists are also represented as working collaboratively, for the common good.

This carries with it a variety of assumptions. Discovery is represented as a single act, and fundamental knowledge is represented as the basis of clinical practice. Tests and treatments are based on applied knowledge, their success depends upon the objectivity and accuracy of the knowledge on which they are based. Genes and disease are represented as stable entities, with respect to the numbers and types of mutations. Even when the range of symptoms and severities of the disease is discussed, the focus is upon an overarching genetic explanation. Difficulties in designing effective testing and treatment are not discussed. This account also strips the local context away from the research process, providing a standardized version of the discovery story, and erasing the role of other actors in the story, including other scientists and clinicians, patients and their families, university administrators, drug companies and regulators. These actors do not appear to have a role in facilitating and interpreting the research as 'a success'.

It would, of course, be churlish to expect the NHGR public relations department to provide a more lengthy and complex sociological analysis of the work of their scientists. Their account is designed to capture attention, to be translated into the popular news, and to encourage fundraisers and supporters of people with CMT and dSMA, in addition to justifying genome research funding. However, we should not take their account at face value.

The scientists involved in discovering the genes involved in CMT and dSMA would have worked in a field which has become increasingly commercialized, even in public sector institutions such as the National Institute of Health. This will shape the focus of their research, the tools and practices that they use and the way in which their work comes to be represented in the public domain. The press release emphasizes the value of chromosome mapping as part of the HGP and suggests, in the words of Francis Collins, that this project is 'accelerating studies in human genetics' – thereby underlining the value of public funding in this area. There have been considerable tensions between the publicly funded HGP and private ventures such as that of Celera, especially around the issue of patenting results. Tellingly, this commercial context is missing from the press release.

A range of other actors involved in the process of discovering *GARS* is also missing from the press release, especially the patients who supplied the materials on which the research would have been based. A range of other ethical and political considerations would have shaped the recruitment of these research subjects, the ways in which they are updated about the progress of the research, and the ways in which these findings are packaged as a step towards finding cures for a variety of patient groups. The politics of genetic research more broadly will also have shaped the way the discovery is represented by the NHGRI and the NIH. It is important to highlight these success stories, thereby underscoring the benefits of genetic research, in a climate where other aspects of work in this field are highly controversial.

The CMT and dSMA scientists will be part of a much wider network of scientists and clinicians with whom they must collaborate and sometimes compete for funding and other resources. This make marketing an important aspect of their work, and brings responsibilities not just to immediate colleagues, but to the institution as a whole. These relationships are absent from the press release, but remain a crucial aspect of the discovery process.

One other set of relationships worth highlighting before we investigate these contexts of discovery in more depth is that between the human and the non-human actors involved in these processes. The functions of tissue, cells and other biological substances associated with these diseases, as well as the package of symptoms which makes up each disease are not simply waiting to be uncovered by the intrepid scientist. Instead, these material and conceptual entities actively shape the process of gene discovery. They make experiments difficult, they contradict assumptions, and they change as they are studied. It is also difficult to link genes to disorders in any clear fashion. Each disorder has a series of subcategories, which involve a range of biological and genetic processes. *GARS* is only implicated in some of these. When we read the press release closely, we see that scientists 'speculate' that a mutation in *GARS* reduces enzyme activity and causes disease, but they do not know how to link this disruption to the actual symptoms of the diseases they are studying. The discovery is still presented as an important step towards cure and treatment.

Knowledge, practice and things

Recent laboratory-based studies in the sociology and anthropology of science have shown how actors construct scientific problems and their solutions in a complex web of relationships between humans and nature. These processes have been shown to be thoroughly social in the sense that they cannot be conceptualized independently of language and discourse. This does not mean that the material world does not exist, just that we cannot assume an Archemedian point of view where what we know is the Truth. Instead, what counts as legitimate knowledge, or truth, is socially negotiated. As Golinski puts it, 'scientific knowledge is a human creation, made with available material and cultural resources, rather than simply the revelation of a natural order that is pre-given and independent of human action' (Golinski, 1998: 6). Materiality and technology obviously play a part in this creation, because they shape how we see the world, but they cannot be disentangled from social relationships. Representations are key to how particular interpretations of events come to be, and multiple, contested versions of the same event are inevitable. There is no straightforward set of relationships between scientists, funding bodies, the press and so on, but a series of fluid relationships whereby each actors' identities are multiple, and their interests contingent upon the particular contexts in which they are placed. The technologies that they produce are equally malleable, and open to a variety of interpretations as they are embedded in different inter-personal, and institutional contexts. According to this analysis, a technology does not have a clear set of values embedded in its fabric, because the intentions of its inventor(s) are far from obvious, stable, or always powerful enough as to be translated into concrete form. Technologies can also become actors in a variety of relationship. There is no straightforward route to the reality of the technologies' effects, because these can only be represented in discourse, and discourses are contested and complex.

Although these analyses are important reminders of the complex layering of social relationships in scientific practice, they have been criticized for taking attention away from the pre-existing structures and power relations that shape technological innovation and design, and for paying little attention to the effects of technologies upon the social world (Kleinman, 1998). It remains the case that some technologies are developed where others are not, and there are important political and economic relationships that shape these developments.

In order to understand discovery in genetics, we need to be mindful of the role and place of the discovery motif in public discourse about genetics as well as the political economies of which it is a part. We need to explore the social and political context in which the processes of discovery are embedded, and the results of which are developed into technologies. This means that we need to consider the funding of genetics, especially its commercial environment, the state's role in sponsoring and regulating genetic research, the genetics communities' values and standards of behaviour, and wider cultural values about differences between people, and the scientific questions which are important. However, we cannot lose sight of the contested and provisional characteristics of genetic research and its effects.

Commercialization

Most contemporary genetic research is conducted in an intensely commercialized environment. Since the late 1980s in particular, there has been a proliferation of biotechnology companies, often founded by geneticists, that conduct various types of research, including gene sequencing at the more 'basic' end of the spectrum and highly targeted research with the aim of developing specific pharmaceutical products at the more applied end. This commercial environment has the effect of further blurring any simple distinction between basic and applied research. Its influence also extends beyond the market place, as it has a significant impact on how publicly funded research is conducted, as we see with the various manoeuvres between the Human Genome Project and Craig Venter's Celera projects over patenting data. On the one hand, research is becoming increasingly centralized through international projects like the HGP which is producing a standardized database, amalgamating the results of thousands of research groups across the world. On the other hand, the commercial environment fosters secrecy and competition between research groups, which makes for a more piecemeal approach to knowledge and technological innovation. This is clearly illustrated in the case of gene patenting, the proliferation of which has shaped the relationships between scientists and clinicians working in similar research areas, particularly in the extent to which they share results and the timing of publications.

Vivien Walsh (2002) provides a useful overview of some of these broad dynamics of biotechnology innovation that also shape genetic research. She notes the rise of the 'network firm', or 'network of alliances and co-operative agreements between a "hub" firm and its partners among smaller specialist firms and in public sector research' (ibid.: 152). The collaborative alliances between producers and user firms, for example in the medical equipment industries, and the growth in joint ventures with firms of similar sizes who share technical and marketing skills, are also highlighted. This has coincided with continual renegotiation of patenting law, so that 'what was once natural and therefore unpatentable has since become patentable' (ibid.: 160). However, the ownership of patents tends not to reflect the multiplicity of actors involved in the process of invention, human and non-human, in terms of organization or location (ibid.: 162). This does not mean that patenting practices are uncontested, indeed a range of groups participate in debates about intellectual property, not just inventors and lawyers, but shareholders and consumers too. On a wider scale still, mergers and alliances are taking place on a transnational scale, and networks are increasingly diffuse, giving biotechnology firms a new flexibility about where and when to produce and market their products. She states,

> The production process of a new drug or crop, from R&D to clinic or supermarket, is becoming increasingly fragmented geographically. Divisionalization of firms is increasingly carried out on a world-wide scale, so that R&D project teams are widely dispersed.
>
> (Walsh, 2002: 170)

Joan Fujimura has studied these processes of exchange of information from the laboratory upwards, and has noted that the wide-ranging networks of which scientists are a part mean that they must represent their work in standard forms, so that they can be easily translated between different settings, This means biological entities like DNA have to be standardized, so that they can become 'codes in the larger arenas of biopolitically universalizing definitions of nature and life' (Fujimura, 1997: 50). Standardization, across laboratories and disciplines also happens through the use of standard databases and software to analyse DNA. These standardizing practices do not simply represent nature in particular ways – they also shape how we conceptualize nature or disease in the future.

The translation of uncertainty is a crucial part of scientific work. For a theory or a technology to be successful, it must be routinized, standardized, easy to transport from one research setting to another. This does not mean that in practice two experiments are ever identical, but that success is marked by the deletion of context, as far as that is possible. Uncertainties do not simply disappear, they are managed or negotiated. One way in which this happens is through the black boxing of technologies or theories, such that their user need not view or understand their inner workings in order to apply them successfully; in other words, their context is deleted. Automation of routine laboratory practices is an important part of this process, as is the wrapping of information into standard packages that can be bought off-the-shelf and given a market value, or biovalue, in Catherine Waldby's terms (2002). This also means that access to information can be restricted to fee-paying customers, through patenting arrangements.

These practices narrow the terrain of what counts as discovery or innovation to a small non-standardized field, putting a spotlight on a limited aspect of scientists' work as other processes become mundane. Gene patenting shapes the process of discovery, in potentially contradictory ways. As we already know, gene patenting is controversial, because of concerns about instrumentalizing life and corporate ownership of parts of people's bodies, but it is also controversial because of its links to discovery. The discovery motif plays a part in the discourse of scientists and corporations who advocate patenting – they see patenting as a means to stimulate and reward discovery and innovation. However, critics of patenting draw a distinction between innovation and discovery, and argue that discovery is an act of uncovering nature, rather than working to produce something novel and worthwhile (typical criteria of patent regulations). They argue that patenting stifles discovery because it restricts research to those who can afford to pay for the right to use patented materials and techniques.

Clearly these processes of black boxing, standardizing and patenting and the discourses and debates around them, have tangible effects upon laboratory practices, even those within the public sector. As Kleinman has argued with respect to laboratory science in the plant biology area:

> Laboratory practice is shaped by the character of agricultural pest control as this field has been defined by a history of industrial dominance, the commercial research supply industry as it has developed following innovations in molecular biology and intellectual property protection, the formal and informal rules and norms that govern the U.S. intellectual property regime, and university-related practices and policies concerning intellectual property protection.
>
> (Kleinman, 1998: 294)

He notes that the agro-chemical industry has been instrumental in defining what it means for a bio-control agent to be effective and how to measure that effectiveness. This shapes laboratory practice indirectly, as the scientists do their work in accordance to what they think is appropriate practice, rather than direct enforcement by the industry. Kleinman also shows how the research-material-supply industry shapes laboratory practice. They produce standardized materials in certain formats. This limits the types of work that is possible, as materials become like black boxes that researchers must take for granted. If the materials are expensive, research is especially limited. Labs may find themselves in difficulties if they try to manufacture the materials in-house, without complying with patents, and their institutions can only offer limited protection against the legal might of multinational corporations should they come into conflict. Of course, researchers also have to consider patenting their own outputs, and this undoubtedly shapes their practices too. Kleinman is not arguing that the researchers are motivated by a drive for personal profit. Instead, he is arguing that they have to foster university–industry links in order to realize the social usefulness of their work, so consideration of patenting becomes inevitable. In his research, the laboratory director used patents to attract commercial interest in the lab work, although she and her colleagues were ambivalent about their implications. These relations are, of course, not set in stone, but they do shape perceptions of what is desirable and what is possible, and this has an impact upon practice in both mundane and profound ways.

Brian Balmer (1996) gives a good example of how these commercial relationships shape the ways in which genes come to be discovered in his study of early mapping work on the HGP. He looked at how two potential styles of research were possible, the 'mapping for mapping's sake' approach which sequenced the entire genome blind, or a more targeted approach that searched for disease genes. Initially, the latter approach was more popular with the British researchers he interviewed, for a variety of reasons. It was seen as more interesting, more publishable and more likely to attract research monies. It fitted into the typical model of peer-review of both grant applications and publications, suiting the needs of journals and funding bodies that emphasized utility, novelty and disease. However, this initial position gradually changed, as the HGP and associated private efforts in competition with it, evolved. Craig Venters' company, Celera, began to patent gene sequences. This meant that the British researchers had to adapt their practices. As Balmer argues,

> A number of distinctions and boundaries were becoming blurred: between basic and applied knowledge; between the reward system of science and the economic reward system; and also the stage at which the genome might cease to be public property. Venter also blurred the boundary between the 'pre-biological' and the 'biological' aspects of genetic mapping. . . . In short, the 'uninteresting' becomes very interesting when viewed from the perspective of industry.
>
> (Balmer, 1996: 547)

Balmer goes on to note that the principal funding body, the Human Genome Mapping Project (HGMP), had to emphasize the novelty of its approach in order to compete with these commercial projects, and to protect their budget from 'raids' by their sister institutions. This meant that they re-oriented their research towards global mapping and the needs of the genome mapping community rather than mapping of particular disease genes. Of course, as Balmer goes on to note, some researchers were able to employ various strategies to blur this boundary and continue their more specific disease-based approach 'on the quiet'. The important point here is that the dominant method and focus of research was fundamentally shaped by both the wider commercial environment and the organizational structure of state funding of scientific research. What counted as a discovery changed from a matter of identifying disease genes, to constructing gene maps.

The scientists involved in discovering the genes involved in CMT and dSMA would have experienced similar constraints on their practice, which would have shaped the focus of their research, the tools and practices they employed, and the translation of their work into a story of discovery. They would have been working with a variety of black boxes and standardized packages of information about the diseases they were studying and the gene functions involved therein. They would have to have been cautious about sharing their results. Their institutions would have taken this need for discretion into account when presenting their results to the press and the scientific community. The protection of patent rights would have shaped these considerations. An emphasis upon novelty and utility in the discovery story is particularly important to prevent commercial companies from patenting similar results.

Governance

National science policy, funding of the HGP and health services, research ethics protocols, particularly constraints on access to patients' records and biological samples, all shape the conduct of genetic research. Regulatory policies concerning research and development, national competitiveness and health provision impact on the type of research that is conducted and the way in which it can be applied. As Herbert Gottweis writes,

> The mainly Western governmental/private efforts in genomics were to a considerable respect responsible for the gradual rise of a broadly based genomics industry with a significant number of new start-up companies involved in a variety of activities.
>
> (Gottweis, 2002: 210)

Government also influences the kind of research that is performed:

> Not only is the boundary between business and academe blurred by definition, there is also a new line of demarcation appearing separating government and academic scientists in large centres able to respond to call for tenders [issued by governmental institutions] and others who are increasingly not part of this new game in biology. The result is not only the shaping of a new industrial/governmental complex, but also a fundamental transformation of biology, far beyond the initial HGP initiative...
>
> (ibid.: 211)

The NHGRI scientists described in our press release are part of this trend, working as they do at a large and prestigious institute – the flagship of the US government's HGP. The large teams involved in the CMT and dSMA research would no doubt have also been working on numerous other projects simultaneously.

Governance nevertheless goes beyond government, and involves a range of professionals, policy makers, patients and publics. Professional standards, audit and ethical review processes in which they are involved shape the structure of research and health care services, as do more informal self-policing within the scientific community to avoid controversial research. Concerns about negative publicity will undoubtedly stifle some research in some laboratories, as might an aversion to lengthy ethical scrutiny and licensing procedures should controversial actors such as embryos, children, or animals be involved. Sarah Franklin illustrates the way in which these concerns shape the process of discovery at the level of the firm and the laboratory, in her discussion of the merger of Geron Bio-Med and the Roslin Institute:

> Geron Bio-Med promises more than smart cell lines and smart venture capital. They are also offering new methods of avoiding many of the

ethical objections to biotechnology by designing life forms that are 'alive' to potential opposition from an anxious or wary public. Until the recent merger, Geron's cell lines came from two sources: human embryonic stem cells (hESs) derived from embryos donated from IVF programs, and human embryonic germ cells (hEGs), which are derived from fetal material obtained from medically-terminated pregnancies. These sources are not only limited, but also morally controversial, especially in the United States, where Geron is based. The merger with Roslin is thus not only desirable in terms of making longer-lasting cell-lines: it is also desirable ethically, which means strategically, because it can eliminate certain controversial aspects of human cell line manufacture.... Whereas eggs, sperm, embryos, and aborted fetal tissue all carry very considerable moral and symbolic weight, and must be donated, it is difficult to imagine organized political or religious objection to culturing a patient's own liver cells to prevent him or her dying of liver failure.

(Franklin, 2001: 340)

In addition to more reflexive professional self-governance, patient groups are also increasingly involved in shaping scientific research priorities, themselves placing strong emphasis on the importance of discovery, in the quest for a cure. Paul Rabinow shows these relationships at work in his study of French DNA (1999). Rabinow draws attention to the creation of new alliances between the different actors involved with biotechnology where value judgements about its morality become 'crystallized'. He shows how the alliance between the Centre d'Etude du Polymorphisme Humain (CEPH) and the Association Français contre les Myopathies (AFM) flourished, in part, because it created a space for public expression about illness and disease. He notes that local values about property, community and national identity also shaped the research agendas and collaborative enterprises of the team of scientists that he studied. This meant that an international alliance, between CEPH and the American biotechnology company Millennium Pharmaceuticals, broke down in the face of disagreement about ownership and access to French DNA.

Returning to patient groups' influence on research, we should note that these groups are often formed by parents or relatives of people who are sick or disabled, in order to raise funds for research and treatment. They have been heavily criticized by organizations of disabled people, who accuse them of being organizations for, rather than organizations of disabled people. However, a range of 'self-help' groups who share interests in promoting research and treatment also exist for people affected by particular conditions, and they too sometimes become involved in shaping scientific research.

Patient and support groups involve a complex mixture of concerns and priorities and their relationships with scientists and clinicians are equally complicated. National differences exist, as do differences depending on the type of condition the group represents. Strong links between professionals and some patient groups can be found in France, as outlined by Volonlona Rabeharisoa and Michel Callon (2002). The patient associations that they surveyed contributed a significant amount of their funds to support research. Rabeharisoa and Callon discuss different types of associations between these groups and medical and scientific professionals. In the auxiliary association model, 'the associations contribute directly to the cost [of knowledge production] in the traditional manner of health care insurance' (Rabeharisoa and Callon, 2002: 61). Alternatively, they might acquire their knowledge and favour certain types of research, becoming 'oppositional' to certain orthodox research. Another model, the partnership association, involves more direct collaboration, where patients' experiences and priorities are taken into account by professionals when negotiating the donation of tissue or good clinical practice, for example, although this is not without controversy.

A range of patient associations in the UK have similar relationships with professionals, sometimes funding research directly through grant-awarding panels with token lay involvement as in the case of the CF Trust, or, as in the case of the Alzheimer's Society Quality Research in Dementia (QRD) programme, taking a lead role in funding decisions. According to their website, at http://www.qrd.alzheimers.org.uk/qrd_advisory_network.htm

> The heart of Quality Research in Dementia is the QRD Advisory network; a network of 150 carers, former carers and people with dementia who play a full role in the following areas:
>
> - They set the strategy for research.
> - They provide comments and prioritization of grant applications.
> - They select applications for funding.
> - They monitor on-going projects being funded by the Society.
> - They tell others about the results of research.

Members of the group are trained on how to assess applications, and award panels are made up of 50 per cent researchers/scientists and 50 per cent members of the QRD Advisory Network. Among the group's priorities for 2002–03 were basic science research into the causes of dementia, epidemiological research on risk factors, genetics research, investigation of triggers for dementia and mechanisms of disease progression, development of new drug treatments, research on prevention, stem cell research into dementia, a cure for Alzheimer's disease, disease modifying therapy, research on diagnosis (early diagnosis, differential diagnosis, diagnostic tests), research on effects of care standards (community care, long-term care, terminal care, care needs and planning), and improving dementia care in primary care.

In a recent focus group with members of this group,[1] their sense of expertise was striking. They made a clear distinction between the uninterested 'person-in-the-street', lacking in knowledge and motivation, and the interest group that they belonged to, borne out of their experiences of caring for people with dementia. One participant noted that as a group they had undergone a process by which they had gained significant knowledge as a result of their involvement in QRD. This same participant also challenged the validity of focus group research and the topics being explored therein, noting their lack of relevance to policy-making.

This suggests that, for this group at least, expertise and citizenship were renegotiated as they took up a role in the governance of scientific and medical research. The authentic experiences of patients and carers and their interests in pragmatic solutions to illness and distress are seen as important drivers of more focused and useful scientific research. This position represents a melding of positivist and interpretivist epistemologies. The group valued the facts of nature and individuals' authentic experiences. Research into the causes of dementia and ways in which it might be cured required both dimensions. The discovery motif remains an important shared discourse for QRD members and professionals alike.

Although there is no mention of patient groups' priorities in the CMT and dSMA press release, they are likely to have played a background role in the support for this research. Other disability activists may have questioned the priority to discover and cure in this case, but for most patient groups this would be uncontroversial. Other aspects of governance, such as professionals' negotiation of the ethics of their research, may also have shaped the kind of discovery stories that are being told. Research into diseases such as CMT and dSMA is relatively uncontroversial compared to work involving embryos or stem cells, or behavioural genetics, for example. It is therefore more likely to be flagged in press releases of this kind. The priorities of the NHGRI, the NIH and ultimately the government will also have influenced the good news story that we see here. The HGP has yet to reap the enormous benefits that were promised prior to the completion of the map, and it is important to cast the successes that have been achieved in terms of these broader aims in order to justify continuing support for this field of research.

Expert relations

Collaboration and competition between scientists, their role in marketing and career building and the hierarchical structure of scientific work also shape genetic research and technological developments. Scientists need to do research into popular topics using up-to-the-minute methods, if they want to get ahead. The identification of disease genes was certainly an important field in the late 1980s and early 1990s, but the extent to which this is still the case is open to question. New areas like pharmacogenomics and stem cell research have probably superseded gene hunting as the cutting-edge research of the moment. It is doubtful whether gene identification would make front-page news as it did a decade ago, now that these newer and in some cases more controversial types of research are also being pursued.

The myth of the lone scientist, or close-knit research group, fiercely competing with other similar groups to discover X, nevertheless remains a potent one. What actually happens between scientists is rather more complex. As

Batchelor *et al.* (1996) have argued, collaboration between scientists and clinicians forms a continuum. It can range between full co-operation, to selective revelations and intense competition. Their relationships are not stable. Crucially, they depend on the stage of the research, changing as knowledge moves from being popular and new to being more established. To establish and build such networks scientists and clinicians must market their ideas and techniques, so that other scientists and clinicians can adopt them too, thereby strengthening the innovator's standing and collaborative links. Marketing is one facet of a wider level of career building that individual scientists, research groups and scientific institutions must engage with in order to maintain and advance their profile in the wider community. Publications must be written and grants secured, or the enterprise halts. Fujimura (1998) calls this 'constructing do-able problems' – setting out the case for research in a particular, novel, area, and being able to deliver.

In the early days of a research field, scientists extend their jurisdiction by creating easy-to-transport techniques and theories that are then adopted by other research groups. Other disciplinary specialities have an interest in these new methods of ideas, because they offer them a route to fruitful collaboration – grant money always flows in the direction of popular, new topics and approaches. Repeated use of these methods or ideas means that they then form their own bandwagon, recruiting other researchers and clinicians who could adapt and apply them in their field.

The line between clinical research and service provision also become blurred as scientists require new clinical subjects and clinicians need to secure research funding and the much-needed clinical and scientific infrastructure that it brings. As I argued previously, the commercial environment also has profound effects on how scientists and clinicians collaborate, especially the extent to which they share information, given the growing use of patents in this sector. As we saw in the previous section, lines between professionals and patients on the basis of expertise are also becoming blurred. These dynamics shape what counts as the 'latest' discovery, and who can lay claim to have had a part in it.

Professional, institutional, national and international collaborations between and among scientists and clinicians mirror their shared interests in particular understandings and approaches to genetic disease. On a local or institutional level, clinicians, scientists and technicians are mutually dependent upon each other to advance treatments, diagnostic protocols and careers. This prompts sharing of patients and clinical material, as well as research results. Shared knowledge and resources at a national and even international level can also be important for all of these reasons. Clinicians' quest for improved diagnosis and treatments and better care for patients and their families with whom they often have long and close relationships must also be recognized as an important motivating factor in their willingness to collaborate with scientific colleagues engaged in basic research.

It is nevertheless important to recognize that this emphasis on mutuality and dependency across geographical, professional and clinical relationships in order to 'discover' the cause of disease, is a discourse in its own right. As suggested earlier, the public relations of genetic disease have become an important aspect of efforts to justify the huge political and scientific investment in genetic research and service provision by the governments of the rich West. The repertoire of collaboration combined with the discovery motif are good selling points. A focus upon scientists' drive to understand, and their competitive instincts is good copy, as is the discourse of clinicians' drive to help their patients suffering from terrible disease. This is reflected in Pam Davies' 1991 article in *The Lancet*, entitled 'Cystic Fibrosis from bench to bedside', which begins

> The highest goal of biomedical bench research is to translate test-tube discoveries into real-world benefits for patients. The extraordinary advances in research on cystic fibrosis in the past 10 years have provided a wealth of opportunities for therapeutic intervention and will surely add new strategies to the current armamentarium.
>
> (Davies, 1991: 575)

The story of discovery can also become part of a wider story of international competition between scientists, as in the so-called 'race to find the CF gene'. The scientific and medical press constructed a compelling story of the international 'race' to find the CF gene as various research groups came closer to its location. Two articles by L. Roberts in *Science* entitled 'The race for the Cystic Fibrosis gene' (8 April 1988) and 'The race for the CF gene nears end' (15 April 1988) in addition to an article by Davies (1990) cast the various groups as intensely competitive, despite their collaborations. Roberts suggested that the British group, headed by Robert Williamson, had not shared an important probe with their competitors, and noted particular disharmony between Robert Williamson and Helen Donis-Keller of US-based Collaborative Research Inc. over commercial involvement in the project. It was also suggested that Williamson's group exaggerated the significance of a candidate gene they had identified in order to stifle their competitors' research funding.

This is an example of a discovery story that was not written by the principal actors in the CF story. Their own versions are rather more nuanced, but still feature talk of collaboration and competition as central to the drive to discover. Lap Chee Tsui, the head of the Canadian group that identified the gene first (in collaboration with US-based colleagues) rationalized their situation thus:

> you want to share information . . . for self-interest . . . because your granting agencies would be looking at your work, ok? Your peers would be looking at your work. So, you had to appear to be ahead of people, right? But as a scientist you don't want to mislead people, so everything you say has to be correct, of course. . . . But then how much [information do] you put out, ok? It's a different matter I think. . . . Self-interest, I think everybody would have that. . . . That's no secret . . . [but there is a] balance [between] how much [information] you keep, and how much you share. And you are

> definitely not sharing everything, yeah, because it kills your fellows, it
> kills your students, because they work so hard too.[2]

For Tsui and others like him, his work is not simply a matter of discovering genes, it also involves a complex series of negotiations around his responsibilities for colleagues, peers, patients, employers and funding bodies. He presented competition as a necessary feature of these negotiations because it stimulates research, but he also argued that it might stifle research if it limited the sharing of information and results. These discourses of collaboration and competition make the case for scientific progress based on a careful balance between mutual respect among CF workers and a natural drive to succeed which provokes competition and rivalry.

The CMT and dSMA scientists are undoubtedly part of their own dense networks of relationships with other scientists, working under similar pressure to secure further funding by producing marketable research, both in terms of actual results, and the techniques that were applied in their construction. They will have obligations to younger researchers within their laboratory, and to other groups within their institution who will also benefit from their fellow scientists' success in the sense that it brings recognition to the institution at which they work. The *GARS* discovery is presented as a justification for sequencing chromosome 7 on which it is located, the major work of the NHGRI team involved in the project. The significance of this work is also underlined when it is used as a justification for further research into a whole suite of neurological disorders, reflecting the interests of the NINDS. Other groups working in similar research areas outside the institution will also have shaped their practice – as colleagues and competitors. This shapes the discourse of discovery presented in the press release, and the focus upon collaboration therein. In other circumstances, we might have found a discourse of discovery linked to competition. We might still find this if we spoke to the scientists directly. However, collaboration and competition are not mutually exclusive – both can clearly feature in the same discovery discourses, depending upon their context.

Defining disease

So far, I have considered the wider context of discovery in terms of their economic, institutional, political and professional contexts. All of these social relations, to varying degrees, shape the discourse of discovery, but when we understand their dynamics we realize that discovery is much more than the simple tale of progress towards enlightenment that they tend to invoke. In this section, I turn to consider another aspect of the discovery process – its relationship to the physical or biological entities to which the discovery pertains. In the case that we have been considering, these entities are diseases, so I will focus upon disease in this section. However, the entity could equally be another biological process, for example the mechanisms of stem cell growth, or the way in which the protein products of genes function within particular kinds of cells. All of these aspects of the biological body are shaped by cultural values and social arrangements, no matter how natural they first appear.

This is easier to see when we focus upon disease, because it is not difficult to grasp that what we call a disease depends upon our culture. For example, infertility is considered by many Western scientists and clinicians to be a disease, yet this is unlikely to be the view of people in the rest of the world. We have come to view infertility as a disease because of our relative affluence and declining birth rate, but also because the technologies of assisted conception which are now available to a much wider population of couples considered to have fertility problems. Conceptualizing these as diseases legitimates the use of the technology in this way.

Paul Martin (1999) has shown that the meaning of genetic disease has also shifted over time. He argues that in the 1970s the notion of genetic disease was re-framed as a common acquired pathology, caused by errors in gene regulation, in response to developments in gene therapy. Gene therapy itself was also redefined from a surgical procedure, to a treatment of inherited disorders, to a drug therapy, as the field developed. These definitions were strategic in the sense that they contributed to the formation of an acceptable research environment, focused upon the discovery and ultimate treatment of the underlying mechanisms of genetic disease.

When we turn to consider genetic disease more generally, attitudes to abortion, personal freedom, autonomy, responsibility for health and disease, and the stigma of disability, alongside increasing medicalization and reproductive surveillance, all shape the types of conditions and impairments that come to be classed as genetic diseases. The way in which particular physical or behavioural conditions come to be considered likely candidates for genetic investigation is a thoroughly social process. Take, for example, obesity. Kaplan (2000) points out that to conceptualize obesity as a disease requires that we view it as in need of medical intervention. Yet, obesity does not inevitably cause health problems, nor is it necessarily the main factor when such problems do occur. Indeed, he refers to some evidence that mild obesity correlates with longer life. Obesity is classed as a major health problem because we live in a society which values thin bodies over fat bodies. These aesthetic considerations have defined obesity, alongside a growing list of physical and behavioural attributes, as diseases. The diet industry has long searched for the magic pill to make us thin. Whether or not genetics will actually provide that remains to be seen. Given that obesity itself involves a range of physical and emotional disorders in some cases, and none at all in others, and that body shape and size are heavily influenced by lifestyle and environment, this is highly unlikely. However, research into the genetic basis of obesity will undoubtedly continue, given the huge financial rewards that are at stake.

Even in what we consider to be the most serious and obvious genetic diseases, like cystic fibrosis, the actual definition of the disease is shaped by biological, material and social processes, rather than simply discovered by careful study of its physical manifestations (see Box 3.2).

Box 3.2 CF History Project – discovering CF

The initial move to define CF as a distinct disease entity was not a unique event, as historical accounts commonly have it, but was accomplished by a series of steps by different researchers. The Swiss paediatrician Guido Fanconi wrote about the familial nature of congenital intestinal obstruction during the 1920s, following in the footsteps of others with an interest in congenital steatorrhoea, including Archibald Garrod who went on to write *Inborn Errors of Metabolism* and Karl Landsteiner, who went on to develop the classification of blood groups. Dorothy Andersen of the New York Babies Hospital, demonstrated in 1938 that the condition that she called cystic fibrosis of the pancreas was not a rare disease. The local conditions of these workers as well as the wider state of medicine shaped their approach to the disease. Andersen, a paediatric pathologist, strove to distinguish CF from Coeliac disease because of clinical priorities – children were not responding to treatment. Her approach to this task was determined by her own specialist knowledge in morbid anatomy, which meant that she focused upon defects in the pancreas when explaining the aetiology of the disease, a point reflected in the name which she gave the disease – cystic fibrosis of the pancreas.

When we track the changing definitions and explanations of what ultimately came to be called cystic fibrosis (although the term muscovidosis is still used in France) there is no straightforward path towards enlightenment. However, there are certain key steps in understanding, such as the move towards conceptualizing CF as a multisystemic disorder (Lowe *et al.*, 1949), the development of the sweat test as a means of diagnosis (Gibson and Cooke, 1959) and the identification of the gene (Rommens *et al.*, 1989). Beyond this fairly flimsy historical framework, there are many variations on the conceptualization of cystic fibrosis, variations that seem, to a large extent, to co-exist without generating huge amounts of controversy. Classic CF corresponded to more serious versions of the disease, but another notion that we could call heterogeneous CF has also existed throughout its history, stressing the variability of the condition, particularly the existence of 'mild' versions of the disease. This is in part a product of the *degree* of difference and variation in notions of the condition. Historically, CF has always been difficult to pin down, so ambiguity about its boundaries is 'normal'.

When it was first conceptualized, CF was usually presented as a fatal illness of childhood characterized by chronic lung infections and digestive abnormalities. Occasional mild or atypical cases were recognized, but not privileged, as the 'unity of the disorder' manifested in abnormal mucous and lesions in the intestine, pancreas, salivary glands, and respiratory system was more important to the contemporary understanding of this relatively new disease category. In the 1950s when the sweat test was developed, the definition of CF changed to include the pancreatic sufficient form of the disease, which could also be diagnosed via this new method. As Barbero and Sibinga argued

> As a result of the knowledge initiated by the discovery of the sweat electrolyte abnormality, the concept of cystic fibrosis of the pancreas has emerged as a familial disease with focal involvement of all the exocrine glands of the body.
>
> (Barbero and Sibinga, 1959: 221)

'Mild' or 'variant' forms of CF also came to be counterposed to classic cases with sweat sodium contents above a certain level. Improving treatments also shaped the understanding of the classic form of the disease. As Kulczycki and MacLeod noted, by 1961,

> the classic pattern of the disease has also changed, since many of the clinical manifestations are conditioned by modern medical care which in many instances prevents or delays the appearance of manifestations or at least ameliorates the severity of the disease.
>
> (Kulczycki and MacLeod, 1961: 85)

Mild or variant cases became particularly interesting in the 1960s and 1970s as work on cell cultures and serum was interpreted as suggesting a heterogeneous genetic effect. Speculation about the possibility of one or more genes being involved in CF can be found throughout the 1980s, as in the review article by Beaudry, where he asks, 'Which gene or genes, can explain all of the above inconsistencies?' (Beaudry, 1987: 5).

The characterization of CF as a classic Mendelian recessive disorder also occurred relatively early in the history of the disease, from the 1950s onwards. CF was often presented as the most common lethal recessive genetic disease in Caucasian populations in the 1960s and 1970s, as statistical evidence of the mutation frequency accumulates. By the 1980s and the 1990s, CF was described as 'one of the most common' (as opposed to *the most* common) 'life-shortening', 'serious' or 'semilethal' (Anonymous, 1979: 626) disease. At the same time, the identification of the CF gene mutation delta F508 in 1989, and the large numbers of mutations found subsequently (now in the region of 1000), meant that discussion about whether or not CF is a clinical continuum or number of related disorders was considerable. In the late 1990s, the 'classic diagnostic triad' of CF (Davis *et al.*, 1996: 1229) still consisted of the 'abnormal sweat test result, pulmonary disease and pancreatic disease' (ibid.) Interestingly, it does not seem that the identification of the gene ever really raised the possibility of a new definition of classic CF on the basis of genotype rather than phenotype. This was largely because genotyping did not simplify the process of CF diagnosis. As Bonnefort and colleagues argued in a 1997 paper,

> Whatever the power of molecular biology, the diagnosis of CF in index cases with a classic phenotype continues to rely primarily on clinical findings and the sweat test. Whether all diagnosed CF patients should be genotyped remains a matter of debate.
>
> (Bonnefort *et al*., 1997: 63)

However, genetic evidence for CF was incorporated into the diagnostic process at a lower level than that of the 'gold standard' (the sweat test). Genotyping also meant that additional features of CF became more prominent in the definition of classic CF. One obvious example, which is extensively discussed in Kerr (2000) is the foregrounding of a form of male infertility as part of classic CF.

These different versions of what I have called classical and heterogeneous versions of CF are not mutually exclusive, nor are they inherently contradictory. Instead, they exist in a necessary tension throughout the history of CF; fuelling further research, refined typologies and diagnostic standards. Their place in the discourse is tied to the technological and clinical arrangements that prompt each contribution to the literature, and they can be mobilized in quite different ways to support a particular argument (e.g. for or against screening). The details of each category are also dynamic, such that 'classical' and 'heterogeneous' can apply to various aspects of CF and its definition – symptoms, severity, or aetiology – and within these categories the relative importance afforded to particular manifestations of the disease varies across time, as knowledge and new technologies develop. Although some workers in the CF field are devoted to a particular version of the disease over another (a paradigm case being that of the clinical geneticist who might dismiss ambiguity about the range and cause of CF as 'noise around the edges' of what is, in their view, a 'fairly straightforward disease'), it is also striking that the dynamic and contextual characteristics of the definition of CF are well recognized, and possibly even viewed as productive, by some scientists in the field.

We often think that diseases are discovered, their underlying cause is discovered, and a cure then becomes possible. However, as this discussion suggests, and the case study of CF illustrates, the links between the conceptualization of disease and its underlying mechanisms are far more complex.

Scientists and clinicians actively construct particular diseases, to promote and justify research in that area. I am not suggesting that they are simply 'making up diseases' because disease clearly has a biological material dimension as well as a social one. This means that diseases are not stable, passive entities, waiting to be uncovered by scientific sleuths. They are highly flexible categories within their own right. The extent to which certain symptoms are considered to be part of a disease, the boundaries between that disease and other similar conditions, the distinction between serious and mild versions of the disease, the identification of the biological processes involved in the manifestation of the disease: all of these things are subject to negotiation among scientists, clinicians and patients. They change over time, not because knowledge evolves in a linear fashion, but because the material, technical and conceptual resources that researchers come into contact with, change over time. This also means that various different notions of disease can co-exist at one time, further complicating the linear picture of discovery and disease.

At this stage, it is also worth mentioning again that the discovery in genetics is not a matter of unearthing little bits of code called genes. The gene itself is ambiguous. It is not simply read off a piece of DNA. To produce a representation of a gene requires several complicated chemical reactions and physical processing. These technologies themselves shape what is seen. This is called instrumentation. This process involves assumptions, amalgams and editing, processes which are then embedded into the genetic representation itself.

The meanings of genes and disease are therefore far from stable, in terms of the symptoms that constitute a disease, the explanation for the disease process and the meaning of disease in relation to future developments. Genes are highly complex, and difficult to understand. So are diseases, which often have a considerable range of symptoms and severities. The CF gene has over 1,000 mutations, and scientists are still looking for more. Each mutation, each subtle alteration in the genetic code, has a unique effect on the protein product. These can be grouped into types of mutation, but there is inevitably overlap in some areas. As research progresses questions have arisen about whether a difference in the genetic code is actually a mutation, or error, or if it is just a difference, with no ill effects. Questions have also arisen about where the CF gene begins and ends. Genes are not simple pieces of code. Understanding their function is also very difficult. Scientists still do not really know what the biochemical processes are which cause CF. This makes it difficult to develop treatments based on gene therapy. They can identify the most common mutations in particular ethnic groups but there is always going to be a level of variation in the types of mutations people can have. This means that rare mutations that are not usually tested for will not show up and some people will not be diagnosed with CF. On the other hand, it is feasible that people who have been diagnosed with CF in its mild form, have been misdiagnosed because the genetic mutation was actually just a difference. These difficulties in testing and treatment contribute to the instability in the meanings of gene and disease.

GARS' relationship to CMT and dSMA is just as complicated as CFTR's relationship to CF. Not only are these disorders linked to other neurological disorders, but they also involve complex subcategories of their own. Different forms of the disease are caused by different patterns of inheritance. *GARS* is only implicated in some of the sub-categories of the diseases, and is also part of a 'gene family', suggesting it is not the only gene to cause these disorders. When we read the press release closely, we see that scientists 'speculate' that a mutation in *GARS* reduces enzyme activity and causes disease, but they do not know how to link this disruption to the actual symptoms of the diseases they are studying. The research is therefore at a very early stage. We can speculate that as knowledge about genes changes, the definition of the diseases will also change. Several versions of disease can exist simultaneously – some emphasizing similarities, others differences in the spectrum of symptoms, for example. Genetic knowledge is not necessarily going to lead to a unified understanding of these diseases, despite the promises of the press release.

Conclusion

As Batchelor and colleagues have argued, discovery is a social process, not a single act (Batchelor *et al.*, 1996).

Genetic discoveries are socially shaped, marked by the politics and social relations that have created them, despite all the work that goes into deleting this context in press releases. Notions of the gene, disease and even testing and therapy are far from fixed. Knowledge, artefacts and practices interface and shape each other. Networks of collaborations between geneticists and their colleagues are also flexible. Crucially, the patterns of flexibility and the management of uncertainty are styled and influenced by the social relations and cultural values of the scientific community and the wider public arena in which they are located. These relationships all affect what counts as a discovery in genetics, and how it is marketed. Standardizaton and black boxing, the patent system and the conflicting pressures of centralization and fragmentation of research activities all shape its outcomes. Professionals' sense of ethics, and their relationships with funding bodies and patient groups also influences their work, and the need to cast it in terms of discovery and progress. This may be linked to a series of collaborations and/or rivalries with fellow scientists and clinicians, but these will only be flagged in press coverage when they are considered newsworthy rather than mundane. Discoveries do not lay bare disease any more than they lay bare scientists' relationships. Rather genes, diseases, and indeed professional jurisdictions, co-evolve in the normal practices of scientific work.

Further reading

Batchelor, C., Parsons, E. and Atkinson, P. (1996) 'The career of a medical discovery', *Qualitative Health Research*, 6: 224–55.

Fujimura, J. (1998) 'The molecular bandwagon in cancer research: where social worlds meet', *Social Problems*, 35: 261–83.

Kerr, A. (2000) '(Re)Constructing genetic disease: the clinical continuum between cystic fibrosis and male infertility', *Social Studies of Science*, 30:6, 847–94.

Martin, P. (1999) 'Genes as drugs: the social shaping of gene therapy and the reconstruction of genetic disease', *Sociology of Health and Illness*, 21:5, 517–38.

4 Reproduction

Summary

This chapter focuses upon reproductive genetic technologies, particularly screening for genetic disease. I begin by considering the dominant discourse in relation to the provision of these services: individual choice. Picking up some of the themes of Chapter 2, I focus upon the ways in which a range of scholars and commentators present these technologies and the values that underpin them in stark contrast to the past. I also note that the focus upon choice at the point of use obscures the processes by which these technologies come to be offered in the first place, and the ways in which they are sustained. Just as the discovery discourse masks the processes by which things are discovered, the individual choice discourse masks the processes by which technologies are designed and implemented. To unpack these processes, I consider the case of Down's syndrome screening in the United Kingdom, looking at who and what has shaped the decision to extend the availability of this form of screening. I end the chapter by considering what shapes women's choices, to complete the picture of the social context of reproductive genetics. I note that their choices are shaped by the clinical circumstances in which they are made, but that women's life experiences are also reflected in their decisions.

Introduction

As I noted in Chapter 2, geneticists and physicians have long sought to prevent the birth of children with genetic disorders. However, it only became possible to terminate affected pregnancies in the 1960s and 1970s, when abortion legislation was liberalized. The identification of these pregnancies also depended upon the development of amniocentesis (to collect foetal cells from the amniotic fluid) and the development of biochemical tests to identify what was initially a small range of chromosomal disorders. Ultrasound screening was used to investigate suspected abnormalities in the foetus or uterine environment in this period. Its use soon extended to all pregnancies, to check for abnormalities in the foetus and to date the pregnancy. Down's syndrome screening came later, in the 1980s, as an addition to alpha fetoprotein screening for neural tube defects, but its provision was patchy and tended to be limited to women considered to be high risk, such as women over 35 years of age. Around the same time, geneticists developed techniques for splicing and cloning DNA that enabled them to investigate genes linked to particular disorders. This so-called 'linkage analysis' developed during the 1980s and 1990s, and was applied in prenatal tests for women with a family history of genetic diseases like cystic fibrosis. These tests were based upon analysis of the DNA in foetal cells, obtained through amniocentesis or chorionic villus sampling. It then became possible to identify particular mutations of various disease genes directly (rather than through linkage) and various mutation kits were developed to perform this task more efficiently. In some cases, these tests grew into screening programmes where they were offered to larger populations than just those families with a history of the disorder. One example of this is the extension of prenatal screening for CF in the United States. However, this expansion has not been as rapid as initially predicted. There is a lack of appetite for these types of ventures in some policy-making quarters. The costs involved in screening for what are comparatively rare disorders, difficulties with choosing the mutations to screen, and problems with predicting the severity of the disease based on these mutations, mean that genetic screening is not as straightforward as many people assume it to be.

Preimplantation genetic diagnosis (PGD) is another new area of reproductive genetics. This was initially developed in the late 1980s as an alternative to prenatal diagnosis, and offered to fertile couples who wished to reduce their risk of passing on a hereditary disease but also wanted to avoid prenatal testing and abortion (Lavery *et al.*, 2002: 2466). PGD involves testing cells from the early human embryo, and the implantation in the womb of embryos that specialists consider to be healthy. However, misdiagnosis can occur, and PGD has been associated with developmental problems and other birth defects, because of a complex range of issues concerning the way the embryo is produced, handled and stored during assisted conception. Concerns have also been raised about embryos being selectively implanted for so-called social reasons, such as sex selection (although this is not licensed in the United Kingdom). Other high profile controversies have involved parents wishing to select embryos whose tissue is compatible with their sibling, in order that they may donate stem cells in order to help with treatment for illnesses such as Fanconi anaemia. PGD is now sometimes also used for infertile couples, to screen embryos for what is called common or age-related aneuploidies, or sporadic chromosomal abnormalities. Leading fertility specialist, Robert Winston cautions:

> Patient desperation, medical hubris and commercial pressures should not be allowed to be the key determining feature in this generation of humans. Bringing a child into the world is the most serious human responsibility. We cannot ignore the clouds lowering over these valuable therapies. To do so could have a profound influence on the progress of medical science, not only in this high profile field, but in others too.
>
> (Winston and Hardy, 2002: s18)

Antenatal screening for genetic disorders is also expanding. In April 2001 the UK Health Minister stated that all women would be offered antenatal screening for Down's syndrome by 2004. This was followed by a recommendation from the National Screening Committee that a national screening programme should be introduced to a basic standard of achieving a 60 per cent detection rate for a 5 per cent false positive rate.

In this chapter, I will begin by exploring the ways in which choice and responsibility are presented in discussions about these various kinds of reproductive genetic technologies. I will argue that individual choice is an important trope in these discussions, and that this has emerged for a number of cultural, professional and political reasons. I will, however, go on to argue that the focus upon reproductive choice, takes attention away from the social context in which these technologies emerge and are sustained. This means that professionals' and policy-makers' choices do not tend to come under scrutiny. When we consider who decides what tests or screening programmes ought to be developed we find that a small group of professionals tend to dominate these processes, and that this masks much of the ambivalence about these technologies which exists amongst those directly involved in service provision – doctors, midwives, counsellors and clients included (Rapp, 2000; Jallinoja, 2001; Williams *et al.*, 2002a,b). As Koch and Stemerding (1994) have pointed out, we also find that these decision-makers are involved in articulating both the demand for the technology and its acceptability, but that these discourses are very limited, dominated as they are by the ideals of technical accuracy and individual choice. The chapter ends with a discussion of the myriad relations that shape women's decision to use reproductive genetic tests. While acknowledging the importance of health care infrastructure and the counselling relationship, I will also argue that women's life experiences shape their decision to participate in reproductive genetic testing, and that this can involve resistance and rejection as well as enthusiasm and compliance.

Reproductive choices

Appeals to reproductive choice are common throughout the medical and ethical literature on reproductive screening. They can also be found in the literature on PGD and prenatal diagnosis, where it is often claimed that these technologies have been developed to meet a patient's need for more reproductive choices. For example, as Braude and colleagues have argued,

> The ability to select an embryo after genetic testing sometimes raises accusations of choosing a child to order, as a commodity that has been designed simply to meet the needs and desires of the parents. This view ignores the fact that most couples make the difficult choice of undergoing PGD as their only hope of a viable pregnancy and of having a healthy child.
>
> (Braude *et al.*, 2002: 946)

The authors also note that, prior to PGD, prenatal diagnosis was available, but that the decision to proceed with this test, with the option of terminating an affected pregnancy, 'was not taken lightly, as termination, especially late in the second trimester, can have substantial psychological and even physical morbidity' (ibid.: 942).

Despite these qualms about late termination, senior genetics professionals often refer to the importance of individual choice when asked about prenatal testing or screening programmes in interview situations. This often takes the form of a default position on which the remainder of their comments rest. Appealing to individual choice can also be a way of deflecting further discussion for those who do not wish to explore its limits. For example, this extract from an interview with a senior geneticist draws a typical distinction between eugenics and genetics on the basis of choice.

> I think my major feeling about that sort of approach to the eugenics question is that we have to keep referring things back to individual choice. I think eugenics for me implies a population, a government, a scientifically led race towards something. I base my practice, and certainly this institution, I'm sure, bases its practice around patient choice. And I think if we aim it at the individual without bias then hopefully we avoid that.
>
> (Kerr *et al.*, 1998a: 193)

Even when these professionals engage in critical questioning of the types of choices on offer, the principle of individual choice tends to remain – as illustrated in Box 4.1.

Box 4.1 CF History Project – interview with two CF specialists: clinician working with adults with CF and molecular geneticist

---

AK: What about antenatal screening for general populations, what do you think of that, as opposed to cascade testing?

1: My own view is that genetically . . . trying to genetically screen a man in the Oxford Road who's never heard of a disease called cystic fibrosis is going to cause so much worry and stress and it's hardly likely to alter his behaviour, my own feeling is it's much better to offer it to anyone in the family, or anyone who wants it. I'm not certain the best use of money is screening whole populations, I know what you think 2.

2: Yes, I totally endorse that and just add yet again the caveat that you . . . can't screen for everything, you cannot fully exclude, OK?

AK: So, for example, we were saying in Edinburgh antenatal screening was available for CF, every pregnant woman's offered it, do you think that's a good idea?

> 1:   I think it's reasonable to allow her to make an informed choice. She's
>   then got to decide whether she wants an abortion or not. And we
>   know the life expectancy of a child born now with CF is forty years.
>
> AK: Do you think that's always properly explained?
>
> 2:   I do think that a lot of the points about CF genetics . . . CF genetics
>   in particular are really quite subtle . . . there've been some studies
>   done, looking at how best to give people information on this kind
>   of thing and how well they understand and retain it. If you give
>   people mailshots, or something written down, then most of them
>   don't look at it, it goes straight in the bin and even if they do look
>   at it, they don't really understand the information. If you actually
>   approach people, you have a healthcare professional approach peo-
>   ple and talk to them for maybe twenty minutes, half an hour, then
>   they understand quite a bit more. However if you go back and ask
>   them simple questions about genetics, about cystic fibrosis a
>   month or so afterwards, most of that information has been forgot-
>   ten, so it needs to be reinforced. So, any kind of counselling sys-
>   tem that you put in place is going to be very costly in terms of
>   personnel and therefore costly in terms of money. So I think that
>   if you open the whole genetic screening game, particularly if you
>   start to involve people who know nothing at all about the disease
>   and don't forget that cystic fibrosis is not the only genetic disease,
>   so if you offer it for CF then you've got to offer it for everything
>   else, then you're opening, in my view, a huge pandora's box
>   and you could spend the whole NHS budget just on genetic
>   counselling, it becomes absurd. So its really a question of how you
>   prioritise this kind of thing.

Although they often express similar concerns, non-specialists also routinely refer to the importance of individual choice in discussions about reproductive genetics. In focus groups with members of the public, the pattern of
their discussions about the acceptability of genetic testing often involves routine appeals to the importance of individual choice. This is followed by some
critical discussion of the current choices and care facilities available to people.
In particular, choice is mentioned when the participants have difficulties
defining acceptable forms of genetic testing (Kerr *et al.*, 1998b,c).

In a more recent study, where scientists with an interest in genetics were
asked to discuss genetic testing for breast cancer, choice was also an important aspect of the process of reasoning. This discussion did not concern antenatal screening initially, although it quickly turned into a discussion of how
testing and screening can develop in this direction, in sometimes unfettered
ways — see Box 4.2.

Box 4.2 'Transformations in Genetic Subjecthood' ESRC Project – Interview, 2002

3: Um as ** has suggested, provided it is done and it's always the choice of the individual.

4: Yes.

3: whether or not to have these tests with the appropriate guidance beforehand as to the implications of having the test, getting the result.

4: Yes.

3: and as long as it is not then going to be passed on to somebody else to identify that individual and potentially refuse them insurance later on.

4: Yes.

5: But it's bound to be asked at the foetus level unless the Government (a) licences the people that do these tests, and bear in mind you'll start to get close to dipstick; you know, dipstick tests which is going to be very difficult to regulate.

3: It's not bound to be asked at the foetus level.

5: Well, but it will be, unless you put controls in, to at least to stop it.

3: These tests are difficult.

4: Ah but I think...

5: They could be...

3: Potentially done...

5: Now, yes, but in a few years' time, it could be very feasible to have these tests done um in Boots, you know. Who would have thought you'd get a cholesterol [test] done 10 or 15 years ago just by walking into Boots, and now you can. So I, I think that's the danger unless you've thought through whether you're going to say there's an absolute blanket [rule] that 'thou shalt not use this test under any circumstances', then you have to regulate who can do the test, how you can buy the kits, and unless you've got that in place in the beginning, and do it worldwide, you're in trouble. Because, you know, the problem is that if you are choosing your eight embryos and you've got no basis to choose them on then why not use the information that's available. Doesn't it make sense? But then would you stop it?

Critics of genetics sometimes also treat choice with special reverence. In their discourses, choice is often referred to as an ideal to which we should strive, even when the difficulties in making free and informed choices are recognized. For example, Bill Albert, a disability rights advocate and member of the Human Genetics Commission wrote in Health Matters in 1999:

> While women should have free reproductive choice, that choice is any-
> thing but free in relation to disability. It is heavily circumscribed by cul-
> tural, social and economic pressures which work powerfully against
> a woman's right to choose to continue with a pregnancy after an 'abnor-
> mality' has been detected.
>
> (Albert, 1999)

This type of appeal to choice is also apparent in the discourses of religious
groups. For example, the Christian Medical Fellowship's submission to the
Nuffield Council on Bioethics' Consultation on Genetic Screening, involved
an appeal to 'holistic' choices:

> We do not believe that genetic screening itself is an evil to be avoided. It
> is a legitimate but limited tool which provides information and it is what
> people do with the information that is important. Society must not see
> abortion as the only solution for those at risk of having affected offspring.
> Genetic screening should be used to allow couples to make informed
> choices with ethically acceptable outcomes (see below). These choices
> should be 'holistic' – ie based on psychological, social, and spiritual
> considerations as well as physical ones.
>
> (Christian Medical Fellowship, 2001)

Similarly, Ruth Hubbard appeals to the need to give people 'real choices'
through challenging the opacity of decision-making about the provision of
antenatal screening (Hubbard, 1997, in Shakespeare, 1999: 679).

Critics also find themselves in agreement with some of the more libertar-
ian bioethicists when they argue that people's choices should extend to the
choice to have a disabled child, as in the recent case of the deaf lesbian couple who actively sought a sperm donor who was deaf so that their child would
be too. Although he clearly disapproves of choosing to have a disabled child,
Savulescu preserves his commitment to choice when he argues that:

> As rational people we should all form our own ideas about what is the
> best life. But to know what is the good life and impose this on others is
> at best overconfidence – at worst arrogance.
>
> (Savulescu, 2002: 773)

Advocates of the most extreme forms of reproductive genetics, such as behavioural enhancement, also appeal to choice. For example, Caplan and colleagues have written:

> In so far as coercion and force are absent and individual choice is allowed
> to hold sway, then presuming fairness in the access to the means of
> enhancing our offsprings' lives it is hard to see what exactly is wrong

with parents choosing to use genetic knowledge to improve the health and well-being of their offspring.

(Caplan *et al.*, 1999: 1284)

Reproductive autonomy and individual choice are also favoured by feminists, who argue that if women have a right to abortion, there can be no differentiation in this right to choose depending on their reasons for wanting to have an abortion. So-called 'social reasons' cannot be better grounds than the reason of 'severe foetal abnormality' (see Sharp and Earle, 2002).

These strong arguments for reproductive choices are difficult to refute, because one is cast as denying women their rights when one raises questions about allowing the elimination of disability, and this apparent denial of women's rights is abhorrent to a lot of people in today's liberal democracies. This is understandable, given the history of eugenics, which is commonly perceived as an exercise in state-sponsored coercion to improve the population. The Nazi excesses of sterilization and euthanasia are a counterpoint to all that today's geneticists seek to achieve: individual choice as opposed to population improvement; the elimination of disease as opposed to the elimination of the feeble-minded (see Kerr *et al.*, 1998a). The atrophy of the state, the rise of consumer culture and individual responsibility for health and well-being, and the extension of civil and social rights to disabled people and women, are all said to mark a definitive break from the past: choice reigns supreme. As Petersen has argued,

> Recent efforts to extend and expand genetic counselling services have occurred during a period in which there has been a radical redefinition of citizenship rights and responsibilities. In the post-welfare era, characterized by the rolling back of state provision of social services and the promotion of an entrepreneurial culture, the emphasis is on the sovereign citizens who is expected ... to take a greater responsibility for managing their own life and relationships.
>
> (Petersen, 1999: 255)

Weaker appeals to reproductive choice, where difficulties in achieving true choice or countervailing pressures to prevent disability are openly acknowledged, are also difficult to challenge, precisely because they are set within a more sophisticated discussion where the limits of choice are clearly acknowledged.

Appeals to individual choice therefore have a role in allowing people to find common ground despite their fundamental divisions over the provision of genetic screening and the elimination of disability. It remains an important ideal, albeit a difficult one to achieve. However, this default position or ideal of freedom of choice has many flaws. As discussed in Chapter 2, our history and our present is much more complex than this story of progress towards individual freedom of choice suggests. Many advocates of voluntary eugenics can be found in the history of eugenics, just as many of today's 'choices' can be considered to be encouraged by the state, through the facilitation of particular social, medical and economic arrangements. As Zygmunt Bauman has argued, choices still have to be confirmed and validated by the market, and one might add, the community, as evident in Rayna Rapp's memorable quote from one interviewee: 'The bottom line is what my neighbor said to me: "Having a 'tard', that's a bummer for life." ' (Rapp, 2000: 91). Choices are necessarily made within social contexts, so the ideal of free, individual choice is a chimera.

This ideal can also have unintended consequences, when it is linked with another contemporary ideal of individual responsibility for health and well-being. The situation of disabled people today is undoubtedly better than that of the past, but they still experience considerable prejudice. Women are often held responsible if they bring defective children into the world. As Barbara Katz Rothman and others have observed, there is a danger that the choice to abort a disabled foetus is an 'impossible choice' which individualizes social problems: 'she chooses, and so we owe her nothing' (Rothman, 1988: 189).

The discourses of choice that can be found in the language of policy reports also tends to sit alongside other less savoury types of analysis, which emphasize the responsibilities of the medical profession and ultimately the state for reducing disabilities – what Abby Lippman calls the public health model (1986). Policy-makers' decisions to proceed with screening on the grounds that it will facilitate individual choice simply does not square with the public health rationale of screening to reduce the burden of disability. As Lippman asks, if women's choices are paramount, why are they not involved in making the decisions about which screening programmes should be developed? Why are all tests not made available instead of being rationed through the NHS? Instead, it is clear that certain choices are more favoured than others. As Angus Clarke puts it:

> An offer of prenatal diagnosis implies a recommendation to accept that offer, which in turn entails a recommendation to terminate a pregnancy if it is found to show any abnormality.
>
> (Clarke, 1991: 1000)

Pointing to this focus upon reducing the burden of disability in policy-making is not to suggest that genetic counsellors or midwives are eugenicists. However, when prenatal screening is offered under time constraints, as part of a broader package of surveillance, people's choices are clearly limited. Although genetics counsellors in particular can be very sensitive to the contradictory rationales for prenatal screening, and are often concerned not to pressurize women into particular courses of action, they deal with a minority of cases (Williams et al., 2002b). Evidence suggests that obstetricians in particular are much less reflexive (Green, 1995).

The important point here is that the rhetorical appeal of individual choice means that these practical constraints on counselling are often not taken seriously when policy-making bodies make the decision to go ahead with screening. This takes place at another level of social organization, beyond the clinic, in the structures of health priorities and budgets, and public health, but it undoubtedly shapes the practices of counsellors and researchers, fuelling their ambivalence and anxieties about their roles (Jallinoja, 2001).

The stress on choice in reproductive genetics also focuses attention on the patient at the point at which the test is offered. As I have just argued, this obscures its political and cultural backdrops, but it also obscures the political economy of reproductive genetics more broadly. There are many layers of investment in the proliferation of these technologies, not in terms of a conspiracy to 'search and destroy' disabled foetuses, but in terms of networks of relationships between researchers, clinicians, funding bodies, manufacturers and academic and medical institutions (Koch and Stemerding, 1994). These groups are all interested in developing new technologies with a bigger return, be it financial or political. The technological imperative is not devoid of humanity, but a product of actors' interests in building careers and laboratories, franchises and footholds in policy networks. The discourse of facilitating pregnant women's choices suits these interests but tends to mask them.

Let us not forget that the discourse of reproductive choice is also an important aspect of the expansion of institutional bioethics – dominated by a range of professional groups with a stake in the governance of reproductive genetics. Bioethics grew after the Second World War, as part of a wider culture of risk management in biomedicine, drawing lawyers, philosophers and theologians into the assessment of the ethics of these new technologies. Bioethics in the United Kingdom has a less clinical tradition than it does in the United States, but its rise is also part of a general opening up of medical practice to outside scrutiny, partly in response to new technologies, such as in vitro fertilization (IVF) and transplantation. Although bioethics involves a range of philosophical and political perspectives, the notions of autonomy and beneficence are some of its central tenets. Context, the province of sociology, is less important. It is therefore understandable that some bioethicists now openly advocate rational reproductive choice as a route to eugenics, and see nothing wrong with efforts to eliminate disability, as we saw earlier. Individual choice is an essentially optimistic discourse, which, as I have previously argued, is difficult to refute. It is a reflection of certain senior bioethicists' roles in policy circles, as acceptably heavyweight counterparts to medical and scientific professionals, whose values and priorities reflect a professional as well as a more general cultural predisposition to support medical progress. Individual choice is an acceptable shared discourse that gives voice to their respective interests in participation in the policy networks.

The narrowing of ethical discussion to unusual cases of prospective technologies, as in the Savalescu paper on procreative autonomy, as discussed previously, is another aspect of bioethical treatments of reproductive genetics. This taste for the bizarre, and somewhat sensational, comes of the philosophical penchant for pushing the boundaries of our thinking through the examination of troubling cases and the drawing of lessons for the more mundane aspects of our morality. This can mean that there is a tendency within bioethics to ignore the subtle 'creep' of reproductive technologies from provision to special cases, to more widespread use for 'at risk' pregnancies, to extension to all pregnant women, as in the case of screening for Down's syndrome or CF.

I do not propose to devote the remainder of this chapter to a discussion of the myriad ways in which individual choices are not purely individual choices, to bolster my argument that individual choice is a myth. I want to avoid setting out an argument that says that we should be aiming for more reproductive choice as a way of countering coercion. Neither do I want to set out a detailed agenda for which reproductive choices women should be prevented from making. This would be to start from the wrong end of the problem, falling into the trap of individualistic thinking, where every question about the rights and wrongs of reproductive genetics has to be reduced to a question of whether or not women should be able to take a particular test.

Instead, I wish to suggest that the focus upon individual choice is itself misplaced, because it masks the professional, economic and political interests around reproductive genetics, and perpetuates the myth that reproductive genetics is inevitably positive. We ought to recognize that the narrow focus on women's choice in reproductive genetics is misplaced and we need to look elsewhere to understand these technologies and their social implications. We need to consider what shapes the development and application of these technologies and shapes women's uptake of them. This involves thinking beyond immediate questions about which technologies ought to be developed or not.

Individual choice cannot always be the trump card, or the way of simply resolving difficult moral issues about what types of people we want to see inhabiting the world. To understand the broader context of reproductive choices we must think about the technological, economic, political and social context of the choices that women are asked to make with respect to reproductive genetics. How do certain technologies come to be developed? Who decides whether or not to implement them on a large scale, and why? How do women experience these technologies?

Down's syndrome screening in the United Kingdom

Since its introduction in the 1980s, Down's syndrome screening in the United Kingdom has evolved in a fairly piecemeal fashion. There is a lack of consistency across health authorities in terms of which types of tests are offered to pregnant women, at what stage in their pregnancy this occurs and the age group that is offered the test (Wald *et al.*, 1998). This situation has been criticized by a number of leading clinicians in the field (e.g. Whittle, 2001), primarily because not all women are offered the Down's syndrome test, and are sometimes offered tests which are not considered to be the best available. Other concerns have been expressed about lack of adequate counselling and the provision of up to date information about Down's syndrome (Williams *et al.*, 2002b).

Equity and informed choice, alongside the increase in litigation against health authorities, are often given as reasons to expand and standardize Down's syndrome screening. However, this is not easy because of a lack of agreement about the best test to use. Disagreements centre around the question of which biochemical markers should be tested, in what combinations, and where the so-called 'cut off' level used to define the population at increased risk of a Down's syndrome affected pregnancy should be located. New screening methods using ultrasound have been introduced, but their value is also contested. A variety of evaluations and audits of these technologies have produced contradictory results.

In April 2001 the UK Health Minister nevertheless stated that all women would be offered antenatal screening for Down's syndrome by 2004, as part of a broad package of improvements to maternity care to standardize services across the country. This was followed by a recommendation from the National Screening Committee (NSC) that a national screening programme should be introduced to a basic standard of achieving a 60 per cent detection rate for a 5 per cent false positive rate. This decision to set standards avoided a difficult decision, about methods but also stimulated considerable debate among the key research teams about the most appropriate methods.

One of the key divisions in the United Kingdom is between a group of researchers who have developed the one stop clinic for risk assessment (OSCAR) (see Box 4.3) and another group lead by Professor Nicholas Wald, which has developed the Integrated Test (see Box 4.4). These groups have been rivals for some time (see Spencer *et al.*, 1992; Wald *et al.*, 1993). They disagree about the markers that should be included, and about the best way of assessing the detection rate of their respective methods (e.g. actual data versus modelling), as well as the benefits and drawbacks of 'on the spot' information versus a delay in providing information and the appropriate uptake rates.

The recent decision of the Antenatal Screening subgroup of the NSC (Box 4.5) to support a menu of screening tests, with the gradual development of the infrastructure and technologies required to support the Integrated Test, means that other tests such as OSCAR (or the combined test, as it is also known) could become established forms of Down's syndrome screening in the United Kingdom as well. The report's emphasis upon 'women's choice' of these tests side-steps some of the economic and political difficulties which would result from a committee such as this advocating the use of only one test. Their decision reflects the gradual evolution of these technologies, facilitated in part by an overlap between research and service provision, that entails de facto entrenchment of these tests without strategic planning on the part of policy-making bodies such as the NSC (see also Koch and Stemerding, 1994). The devolved structure of UK health care has meant that a range of different services have evolved in tandem, and that each of these has depended upon the priorities of local providers, scientists and clinicians with an interest in particular screening technologies. The emphasis upon a range of tests also reflects the relationships between innovators, policy-making bodies, their scientific

Box 4.3 OSCAR

The One Stop Clinic for Assessment of Risk (OSCAR) uses a combination of blood tests of biochemical markers (free β-hCG and PAPP-A) and ultrasound assessment of nuchal translucency (NT) in the first trimester of pregnancy (10–13 weeks).

OSCAR was developed by researchers in three centres in the United Kingdom: the King's College Hospital and the Fetal Medicine Centre (FMC), both in London, and Harold Wood Hospital, Essex. It is currently available to the general antenatal population at Harold Wood Hospital. The FMC organize an accreditation scheme for the nuchal translucency thickness screening – The Fetal Medicine Foundation Certificate of Competence. Charges are made for accreditation (except where this is part of a research study) with profits going towards the support of a charitable foundation outside of the NHS. OSCAR is prompted on the basis that:

> Screening for chromosomal defects in the first rather than the second trimester provides earlier reassurance for those with a normal result and less traumatic termination for those choosing this option.
>
> (Bindra *et al*., 2002: 224)

The researchers argue that healthcare planners' decisions about the viability of this screening programme should not simply be based on cost benefit analyses. Indeed they argue that this would be 'contrary to the basic principle of informed consent':

> Our responsibility is to assess the risk of a pregnancy being affected using the most accurate method and allow the parents to decide for themselves for or against screening.
>
> (ibid.)

Based on a number of studies, the detection rate of OSCAR for a 5 per cent false positive rate lies somewhere between 92 and 96 per cent (Spencer *et al*., 2003).

advisors and the pharmaceutical companies who supply reagents and testing equipment to the NHS. As Lippman observes '[Choice] is increasingly translated into a multiple-choice menu to support the privatization of health (care) and the growth of health industries' (Lippman, 1999a: 282). A range of stakeholders will be able to benefit from the proposed arrangements for Down's syndrome screening in the United Kingdom. This includes the organizations

Box 4.4 The Integrated Test

The Integrated Test, combines information from a biochemical marker (PAPP-A) identified in a blood test with a neural tube (NT) measurement performed using ultrasound in the first trimester and the quadruple blood test in the second trimester (which tests for AFP, unconjugated oestriol uE_3, free β-hCG (or total hCG) and inhibin-A).

The lead advocate of the Integrated Test, Nicholas Wald, recently headed a multicentre research project into 'First and second trimester antenatal screening for Down's syndrome', commissioned by the Health Technology Assessment programme, which is known as SURUSS – Serum, Urine and Ultrasound Screening Study (2003). The HTA programme is part of the National Health Service research and development programme, and is tasked with ensuring that 'high-quality research information on the costs, effectiveness and broader impact of health technologies is produced in the most efficient way for those who use, manage and provide care in the NHS'. The SURUSS study concluded that the integrated test offered the most effective and safe method of screening, followed by the serum Integrated Test if an NT measurement was not available, the quadruple test, and, finally, the combined test (also known as OSCAR). Wald and colleagues concluded:

> The SURUSS results show that in antenatal screening for Down's syndrome it is now possible to obtain a high level of detection (detecting 8 or 9 out of every 10 affected pregnancies) with a false positive rate (1–2 per cent) that is substantially lower than in the past, so achieving a significantly higher level of safety by reducing the numbers of women who need an invasive diagnostic test such as amniocentesis.
>
> (Wald *et al.*, 2003: 49)

The SURUSS report notes that Wald is a director of Intema Ltd which holds a patent application on the integrated test. He is also director of Logical Medical Systems Ltd, which produces alpha^{TM} a commercial interpretive software package for Down's syndrome screening using ultrasound and serum markers. Various companies provided free reagents to the SURUSS study, including Perkin Elemer Life Sciences (Cambridge, UK) who provided reagents for the AFP, uE_3, free β-hCG, total hCG and PAPP-A assays and Oxford Bio-innovation and Diagnostic Systems Laboratories Incorporated (Oxford, UK) which provided the reagents for the inhibin-A assay.

Box 4.5 The Antenatal Screening subgroup of the UK National Screening Committee

---

The Antenatal Screening subgroup advises the National Screening Committee on the implementation, development, review, modification, and where necessary, the cessation of antenatal screening programmes. The subgroup is chaired by Prof Martin Whittle. Nicholas Wald is also an honorary member/scientific advisor.

The Antenatal Screening subgroup has produced a report entitled 'Antenatal screening for Down's Syndrome – National Guidance on Policy and Quality Management' (2003), where it argued that women ought to choose which test they would prefer – so, for example, the combined test might be chosen by women who book for antenatal care in the first trimester and are prepared to make a decision based on the result of the combined test; and the integrated test might be considered appropriate by women who preferred to wait until they had the results of the combined test and the quadruple test. The group favours the integrated test, on the basis that this has the best detection rate and lowest possible false positive rate, but recognizes that various other tests have a good detection rate and that 'Down's syndrome screening should be offered as a programme, and not a single test'. The NSC will commission suppliers of NT screening and inhibin-A equipment and reagents as part of the process of implementing a national screening programme.

---

that are contracted to provide training and accreditation for the uses of these technologies, as well as the analytical software, testing equipment and chemical reagents. This also includes the professionals with a stake in managing and co-ordinating screening services, some of whom are already well-placed entrepreneurs in their own right.

The NSC decision and the reports on which it is based are dominated by technical considerations of the acceptability of these various screening practices. These considerations reflect the views of scientists and clinicians who co-ordinate antenatal services, rather than the views of many of the health professionals who are directly involved in their provision, or indeed the pregnant women to whom they are offered. Although reproductive choice is a prominent discourse, it is articulated by a narrow range of professionals, who act on behalf of pregnant women. Reproductive choice is a flexible discourse, which is used to support particular professional and policy positions. This can mean that authors emphasize a lack of reproductive choice in order to criticize particular screening tests. For example, concerns might be expressed about high levels of compliance with one test – Whittle (2001) raises concerns about the 97.6 per cent uptake of the combined test in one study. In other situations, reproductive choice is not so prominent a concern.

For example, the antenatal screening group report bases its calculations of the efficacy of screening on the assumption that 80 per cent of women offered a Down's syndrome screening test would accept the offer, without considering what this might indicate about the extent to which women are making informed choices about their participation.

Appeals to reproductive choice can also mean that policy-makers avoid having to make a clear choice between particular technologies, a choice that is presented as being left to individual pregnant women. This implies a transfer of responsibility away from service providers to clients, and raises questions about the sense of obligation that this might engender in pregnant women faced with such a choice. Little or no consideration is given to how to facilitate women's choices in practice. Imagine women presented with a menu of possible Down's syndrome screening tests. Were this even possible (and this seems unlikely, given that many health authorities do not even offer one of the preferred tests), engaging with such a menu is hardly a straightforward choice. This range of options could cause confusion and anxiety. It could increase pressure on women to comply, partly because viewing a menu suggests that a choice not to partake is unreasonable, and partly because already overstretched midwives will find it difficult to provide a detailed discussion of the pros and cons of these various tests, and end up taking the easy route of recommending a particular test. Many similar studies have demonstrated that within these types of context, individual women do not make autonomous choices. As Marteau and Croyle have noted, there is some evidence that high uptake rates are also associated with decisions based on less information (Marteau and Croyle, 1998: 693). Others have noted that the lack of information and counselling provided to ethnic minorities is associated with higher rates of compliance with testing (Holtzman and Shapiro, 1998). Yet, the antenatal subgroup report and the SURUSS evaluation do not address these concerns about routinization of Down's syndrome screening, concerns that are often expressed by genetic counsellors and midwives. As Lippman puts it, ' "needs" for prenatal diagnosis are being created simultaneously with refinements and extensions of testing techniques themselves' (Lippman, 1991: 33).

The focus upon efficacy and acceptability also takes attention away from the quality of the information that is provided to pregnant women regarding Down's syndrome. It is somewhat ironic that, at a time when much is being done to tackle discrimination against people with Down's syndrome, a nationwide screening programme is being established to prevent the birth of children with the condition. Many health professionals and associated colleagues are ambivalent about Down's syndrome screening – including members of research ethics committees (Reynolds, 2003). Practitioners also acknowledge that the way in which Down's syndrome is presented affects uptake. A negative picture of Down's syndrome, which does not acknowledge that proper treatment and early intervention can improve the prognosis for affected children, is likely to increase the uptake of the test (Williams *et al.*, 2002a,b). In Brunger and Lippman's study of genetic counselling for Down's syndrome, they found that, 'in contrast to the one-size-fits-all genetic counselling model . . . information transfer is actually custom-made, with the ideas about Down's syndrome and prenatal testing held by both counselees and counsellors shaping, and shaped by each other' (Brunger and Lippman, 1995: 164). This co-production of genetic knowledge can mean that counsellors anticipate what they perceive to be clients' needs and wants, and inadvertently lead them towards decisions reflecting these priorities.

The stakeholders involved in deciding what kinds of Down's syndrome screening programmes are developed have particular reasons for promoting certain tests. However, these reasons are largely hidden from view. Just as the claimed benefits of screening for clients tend not to be unpacked, the financial and political benefits to the professionals and companies who influence policy-making and service provision are largely hidden from outside scrutiny. In contrast, midwives and other health practitioners who are directly involved in service provision, disabled people, the organizations that represent them, and their carers, are not well represented in these policy networks. Nor are the women in whose interests the screening programme is apparently being implemented.

Screening programmes with little time for intensive counselling also seem to pay scant regard to the values and perspectives that clients bring to the clinic. Their attitudes to disease are rarely explored, so the stigma of diseases like Down's can remain unchallenged. Certain groups of women appear to be more compliant with testing without necessarily engaging with its risks and benefits. As Rapp puts it:

> women's socio-economic class standing, especially as it determines the neighborhoods in which she and her family live, and the areas surrounding the hospital that will serve them, has already shaped prior health experiences and the feelings of trust or mistrust with which a pregnant woman undertakes a counselling appointment. A woman's comfort or discomfort with the scientific worldview and language is also deeply affected by her class-based experiences, especially, but not exclusively, through education.
>
> (Rapp in Rothenberg and Thomson, 1994: 222)

Rapp's point here is that we must first think about women's experiences if we wish to understand their decisions, rather than simplistic categories of class. She continues that stereotypes of race are just as damaging as stereotypes of class, when trying to understand what influences people's decisions to take a genetic test. What is important is what Rapp has called people's 'culturally specific, historical legacies', which meld social structure and individual, personal biography.

Reproductive and life history are other obvious mediators in decision-making about genetic testing. People's decisions about antenatal testing will obviously depend upon the number of other children they might have, the support network available to them should their child be disabled, and so on. Although we might expect that if a couple already has a child with a genetic disability they might be more likely to have a genetic test and abort if it were positive, there is some evidence that the opposite effect occurs. A small British study of testing by expectant couples who already had children with CF revealed low levels of uptake, with 17 per cent rejecting any counselling. When prenatal testing was offered, it was declined by 75 per cent of parents and a positive prenatal test was not followed by abortion in the remainder (Lane *et al.*, 1997). On the other hand, the less support people have in caring for disabled people the more difficult it can be to contemplate bringing another disabled child into the world.

A whole range of cultural and social relations encompasses any one decision about genetic testing. People's pre-existing understandings of heredity, as well as wider knowledge of the methodologies, institutions and cultures of science and medicine mediate their responses to genetic testing. They may consider genetic testing to be a means of gaining further information, to empower them in their future health decision-making, or it may add to an already heavy sense of fatalism about their genetic futures. Genetic testing may be experienced as an intrusion, an unwelcome form of surveillance, or as a health right. Women's pregnancies may be tentative as Rothman (1988) puts it, or embodied. They may have a strong connection to their unborn child, or a sense of its fragility and open future. Their notions of genetic responsibility, to their unborn child, other kin and even society at large, as well as their religious beliefs and values, will also shape their attitudes to genetic testing.

Genetic information has various meanings, which can coexist or contradict, depending on each person's experiences and attitudes. As Parsons and Atkinson have argued, drawing on their study of 'lay constructions of genetic risk' in a group of women who were tested to see if they were carriers for Duchenne muscular dystrophy, 'The majority of women...had translated their risk liability into everyday recipes for reproductive action that could be incorporated readily into their personal stocks of knowledge' (Parsons and Atkinson, 1992: 454). Risks are not disembodied facts and figures but they are socially constructed and socially mediated, in the sense that people's interpretations of their genetic risks are embedded in their pre-existing life worlds. Thinking about genetic risks this way helps us to understand why people may or may not choose to take a genetic test, and what they then do with the information it brings. Rapp sums this up well, with respect to prenatal testing,

> Each pregnant woman brings the light and shadow of her personal biography, family history, and community resources, as she hears about new or partly new interventions into her aspirations for her own and her child's futures through these filters.
>
> (Rapp, 2000: 77)

Unfortunately, screening programmes do not tend to give women or health professionals the opportunity to explore these aspects of identity and how they might influence their decision to participate or not because of lack of time for counselling.

Conclusion

I began this chapter with an exploration of the ways in which the discourse of individual choice is mobilized in discussions about reproductive genetics. Choice marks modern genetics as distinct from the eugenics of the past. Choice is represented in terms of patients' demand for these technologies, and as such is very much a part of the consumerist ethos of modern medicine. Although doubts are expressed by many about the extent to which people's reproductive choices are free and fully informed, there is little appetite for the argument that choices should be curtailed. Choice is therefore an important discourse for proponents and critics of genetics alike. As such it forms a useful bridge between their discussions – which might otherwise be far too distinct for any meaningful dialogue to take place.

Such dialogue reflects and supports institutional reflexivity among a range of professionals involved with reproductive genetics, many of who are sceptical about widespread use of the technology, particularly in screening programmes which target populations rather than individuals. However, a range of institutional and governmental actors are engaged in extending these programmes in order to standardize service provision across the country. There is some engagement with the critique of choice when these policy communities focus upon minimizing coercion, but individual choice is more usually mobilized as a reason to proceed with screening, not a reason to deny women these services.

Choice, however, has its own tyrannies, when it involves clients digesting complex information in an atmosphere of anxiety. When professionals give clients choices they also give them responsibilities for those choices, which can be burdens in their own right. In many ways, this version of choice privatizes responsibilities for preventing disability, or, should the test be declined, facing up to the future of living with a disabled child. Women's main choice is to take up or reject the test. Other forms of engagement with these technologies are fairly unusual. Some affected families work closely with clinicians to develop prenatal diagnostic tests for their genetic disorder. More usually, clients have little input into the design and development of these technologies, particularly where screening is concerned. The focus upon individual choice at the point of use masks the many professional choices which determine which screening programmes are established and why. A range of material, commercial, professional and bureaucratic actors shape the design and implementation of these technologies, from the broad aims of the programme of which they are a part, to the fine details of which tests to use, and error margins to accept. As Koch and Stemerding have argued, these technologies are prone to entrenchment in the health care service – once developed they are difficult to displace.

Paradoxically, the very screening programmes which are promoted on the basis that they will extend choices to more women can actually reduce them. When counselling is cursory, choices are too. When counsellors do not have time or the inclination to explore the things that influence their clients' decision with them, there are not many opportunities for informed and reflexive choices. Women's opportunities to exercise the choice to refuse the test are also curtailed. We cannot say that such screening programmes automatically reinforce prejudice against people already affected by the conditions they are designed to eradicate. There is little empirical evidence for such claims. It would nevertheless be too simple to argue that these programmes are entirely divorced from social attitudes to disability, as they are obviously influenced by negative portrayals of conditions like Down's syndrome. Why else would they be designed to prevent them? As Clarke (1991) has argued, because these screening programmes reflect negative values about disability, they can tacitly reinforce them. However, women who participate in genetic counselling concerning reproductive genetic testing and women offered genetic screening, bring a range of experiences to these encounters, which means that their choices are not necessarily foregone conclusions. Some women choose to take up these services on the basis that they would not abort an affected foetus, but prepare for its arrival. Others refuse to be tested because of particular beliefs about disability or termination. Women who decide to proceed with testing often do so after intense contemplation of their circumstances and values. Although these aspects of choice tend to be ignored when large-scale screening is introduced, they are important ways in which women recast institutional choices to make them their own.

Further reading

Koch, L. and Stemerding, D. (1994) 'The sociology of entrenchment: a cystic fibrosis test for everyone?', *Social Science and Medicine*, 39:9, 1211–20.

Lippman, A. (1999) 'Prenatal diagnosis', *American Journal of Public Health*, 89:10, 1592.

Rapp, R. (2000) *Testing Women, Testing the Fetus, the Social Impact of Amniocentesis in America*, New York: Routledge.

Williams, C., Alderson, P. and Farsides, B. (2002b) 'Too many choices? Hospital and community staff reflect on the future of prenatal screening', *Social Science and Medicine*, 55: 743–53.

5 Patients

Summary

In this chapter, I will review the research on patients' experiences of genetic disease, exploring the various ways in which patients, families and professionals are constructed therein. I will consider a range of different approaches, from the more psychosocial approach of medical professionals, to the various strands of research in medical sociology, focusing upon biography and narrative, especially work which concerns strategies for 'coping' with and managing risk and responsibility, and patients' own representations of their experiences in academic texts. Although I will argue that this work gives both rich and sophisticated insight into patients' and their families' experiences, focusing upon patients has its drawbacks as well as its advantages.

Introduction

Research into the social aspects of genetics is dominated by a focus upon patients' and their families' perspectives and experiences. There exists a broad swathe of empirical evidence concerning the illness narratives and coping strategies of people affected by a wide variety of genetic disease. Researchers have looked at people's experiences of late-onset disorders such as hereditary breast and ovarian cancer (Hallowell and Richards, 1997; Rothman, 1998; Finkler, 2000; Hallowell and Lawton, 2002) and Huntington's disease (HD) (Cox and McKellin, 1999; Novas and Rose, 2000), and genetic diseases which affect people from birth, notably CF (Stockdale, 1999; Chapman, 2002; Lowton and Gabe, 2003), and Sickle-cell disease (Atkin et al., 1998). Other work on women's experience of prenatal diagnosis (Rapp, 2000; Marteau and Dormandy, 2001) and preimplantation genetic diagnosis (Lavery et al., 2002; Franklin and Roberts, 2001) has provided a rich source of data on the ways in which genetic diseases impact upon people's lives. A different, but related cadre of work comes from scholars in disability studies, who have drawn from their own experiences of what it is like to live with a genetic disease to present a more positive picture (Shakespeare, 1995; Parens and Asch, 2000), while at the same time criticizing their positioning as 'patients', because of its overtones of passivity and dependency.

The psychosocial model of health and illness foregrounds patients' and families' suffering and distress. This type of research is often conducted by health professionals in collaboration with social scientists. Patient's responses to their illness are linked to psychological barriers to acceptance, such as denial or fatalism. The task of medical professionals is to encourage them to adapt to their new conditions, and comply with treatment. This paints patients as victims, first of their disease, and second, of their mind. Their treatment by the medical profession, and the shifting and sometimes contradictory ways in which they experience their illness, are of less interest.

Researchers from a more sociological tradition tend to take a more holistic approach, focusing upon people's experiences of stigma and discrimination and the ways in which they cope with uncertainties about their condition. This work is often based on in-depth qualitative interviewing, and as Julia Lawton has argued, 'has served to champion patient's perspectives by placing them centre-stage' (Lawton, 2003: 25). Sociological work on lay experiences of illness extends our understanding of suffering from a largely medical conceptualization to one rooted in an understanding of the daily contexts of people's lives. This empirical work draws from and supports a more theoretical orientation to the ways in which people's accounts of illness are stories about themselves, for example, about the ways in which chronic illness 'disrupt' their biography, as outlined by Bury (1982) or the experience of 'loss of self' (Charmaz, 1983). As Lawton notes, another influential theory has been that of narrative reconstruction, as advanced by Gareth Williams (1984). Williams notes that people use a range of concepts to give an account of the meaning of their illness, not so much as a form of disruption, but as part of a broader continuum of experience, which gives disease a legitimate place within their lives. This theme has since been followed up by numerous medical sociologists, concerned with a more symmetrical approach to people's experiences of illness, which looks at the negative and the positive aspects of their strategies for dealing with disease. Others, including Bury (2001) have taken up an interest in how people construct accounts of their illnesses and experiences in particular contexts, looking at how our stories about who we are, and where we came from, are flexible constructions, characteristic of reflexive modernity (see Lawton, 2003 for more thorough discussion).

We can find all of these types of analysis in research on patients' and families' experiences of genetic diseases. Particular emphasis has been placed on the ways in which genetic information and treatments generate new forms of responsibility for oneself and one's kin. Kaja Finkler has studied the ways in which women responded to a diagnosis of hereditary breast cancer, arguing that this has 'medicalized' family and kinship (Finkler *et al.*, 2003). Carlos Novas and Nicholas Rose have drawn from the web-based accounts of people, in families affected by HD, to argue that genetic information about their condition transforms people's relationships in sometimes unexpected ways. Hallowell and Lawton have argued, with respect to women considering prophylactic surgery in order to manage their risk of hereditary ovarian cancer, that they are ambivalent about the extent to which these technologies give them control over their bodies and future identities (Hallowell and Lawton, 2002).

However, there remains a problem with this focus upon patients' experiences of genetic disease. Much of the research in this area aims to understand how patients experience these new technologies in order to improve their provision. This takes attention away from the practices of professionals and the question of whether or not the technologies should be available in the first place. The focus upon patients' attitudes to their health and illness, their uptake of testing, and their family relations, takes attention away from their engagement with support groups and charities, people within their communities and workplace, as well as policy-making bodies, politicians and academics studying their experiences.

This focus upon coping with and experiencing genetic diseases within the family also tends to position other family members as honorary patients, especially since the hereditary nature of genetic disorders has implications for other family members' risk status. As many sociologists have noted, this extends the status of patient to presymptomatic patients, who are conceptualized as people waiting to become ill. This reflects a wider trend in contemporary society to pathologize a growing list of health behaviours and lifestyles. This extension of patient status also takes attention away from the wider contexts of people's lives, and the ways in which they resist the challenge of the biomedical and psychosocial aspects of illness and hereditary risk. I now explore each of these areas in turn.

The psychosocial approach

The psychosocial approach to families with children affected by genetic diseases comes from a tradition in which it was assumed that the birth of a disabled child, or the diagnosis of a genetic disease, was a tragedy for affected individuals and their families. This has long been the view of medical and associated professionals, even those who rejected the extremes of eugenics. As Ferguson and colleagues have shown in an impressive historical review of family research, the impression that these births are the fault of the parents abated in the mid-twentieth century, as eugenics fell out of favour. However:

> Professionals now shifted their attention to how disabled children inevitably damaged the families to which they were born. Whether they preferred to use primarily attitudinal categories (guilt, denial, displaced anger, grief) or behavioural ones (role disruption, marital cohesiveness, social withdrawal), most researchers assumed a connection that was both intrinsic and harmful to the parent-child dyad.
>
> (Ferguson *et al.*, 2000: 76)

Ferguson and colleagues go on to give several examples of the conclusions of this kind of work. If families were unhappy with the health professionals dealing with their case, researchers labelled this displaced anger. If parents did not challenge poor services, they were said to be experiencing guilt or denial. This type of formulation is well characterized by one extract from a paper entitled 'Parentalplegia' from which Ferguson and colleagues quote, and I reproduce below:

> Children having conditions of mental retardation or other handicaps involving physical deficiencies are likely to be causes of a secondary handicapping condition involving the parents. . . . The authors have chosen the term parentalplegia to describe a secondary psycho-physiological (stress inducing) condition that evolves among parents of handicapped children. Parentalplegia seems to be caused by an inability on the part of parents to adjust to the handicap of their children.
>
> (Ferguson *et al.*, 2000: 78, quoting Murray and Cornell, 1981: 201)

Ferguson and colleagues sum up this genre thus: 'Apathetic or involved, angry or accepting: there was a professional explanation of the pathology behind any conceivable parental response' (ibid.: 77).

Although Ferguson and colleagues go on to argue that family research has since changed, we can still find echoes of this psychosocial approach in the literature on families' experiences of genetic diseases. Professional research into services and support for people affected by genetic diseases often focuses upon the burden of the disease, at times implying that this flows from the physical and mental impairments of the infant, rather than the lack of social support for their care, as in the following extract:

> An increasing number of children with cystic fibrosis are now living to adulthood as a result of early diagnosis and intensive treatment . . . Heart and lung transplants are increasingly an option for some. . . . Thus families have to endure this burden of caring for a protracted period of time. In these circumstances many families exhibit evidence of the psychological, physical and financial burden under which they are living.
>
> (Coyne, 1997: 122)

Although there are undoubtedly difficulties for families in these situations, this equation of longevity with burden of caring is exceedingly pessimistic. The emphasis upon supporting families also tends to infantilize adults with CF by focusing upon their dependency on their families and health professionals. Other similar studies have focused upon the 'maternal adjustment' in mothers of children and adolescents with CF and sickle-cell disease, noting the effects of illness severity, and child psychological adjustment among other factors (Thompson *et al.*, 1994). This suggests a causal link between parental psychological function and the biological and psychological function of their child and suggests that parents must adapt to their child's pathology. Such an analysis 'biologizes' the highly social and variable process of intimacy, dependency and distancing that characterize relationships between parents and their children.

Although this type of research often goes on to stress the need for improved support, the rooting of the problem in the child's impairment goes largely unquestioned. Health professionals' anecdotes about marital disharmony and break-ups among families caring for children affected by genetic disorders reflect this too. The problems of family life are often seen as resulting from the impairment, rather than social arrangements, as is suggested in the following extract:

> When a child has an increased risk to health or development, parents must reckon with very personal feelings of anxiety, and in some cases of grief and loss, while simultaneously attending to the special needs of the child. Mutual support by the parents for each other – and other family members – not uncommonly takes a back seat. A familiar pattern in these circumstances is for one parent to become fully dedicated to the ill or disabled child while the partner, often the father, takes a more distant and peripheral position. When this pattern persists and becomes more entrenched, feelings of neglect and lack of support may be experienced by one or both parents. Feelings of resentment toward the child may emerge. It is not uncommon for pediatricians to hear from the main caretaking parent after the break up with the spouse that taking care of the child is 'simply easier this way'. Parental separation and divorce: can we provide an ounce of prevention?
>
> (Tanner, 2002: 2)

Children's pathological response to the burden of their disease is also emphasized in research into their experiences. For example, one study concluded that children with CF have higher levels of 'internalizing symptoms' (such as worries, poor self image and anxiety), than healthy control subjects (Thompson *et al.*, 1990). These children's reactions to stigma or discrimination were framed as if they were symptoms of the disease, rather than responses to negative social arrangements and cultural values.

Even work that presents a more holistic analysis of parents' and disabled people's experiences reflects this medical approach. For example, a focus upon people's 'emotional responses' or 'internal striving' (Larson, 1998) in relation to disease, takes attention away from their social circumstances. The focus upon the individual in psychosocial research also takes attention away from the broader social arrangements which shape the way that families deal with disabled children, reflected in statements such as 'coping with a physically or intellectually disabled child is a highly individual process' (Taanila *et al.*, 2002: 73). Interpreting people's accounts of their health problems as being unrelated to their disease as a form of 'denial' (Lowton and Gabe, 2003) also suggests a pathological psychological response to their truth of their impairment. This takes little account of how people's relationships to their impairment, and how they account for its place in their life at any one time, are dependent upon their broader social context.

Nowadays there is much more emphasis on the need to support and provide services to individuals and families affected by genetic diseases. It is now recognized that these services are not just a response to the physical manifestation of the disease, but that people's experiences of the disease must also be taken into account when planning and providing services. However, the assumption that people's troubles flow from physical impairment, as opposed to social barriers to equality, remains implicit in a lot of contemporary work on patients' and their families' experiences of genetic diseases. It is clear that much of this type of work has been influenced by a biomedical view of diseases, even when it does not directly emanate from this domain. Here, physical and mental attributes are biological rather than social phenomena, and disease is a pathology that people instinctively seek to avoid or minimize (unless, of course, they are ill in another way). Doctors, of course, have easy access to patients and therefore research subjects. Given that they already hold a position of a knowledgeable expert in relation to deviant biological processes, it is not difficult to apply the same methodology to the study of aberrant psychological processes. Psychologists from a more cognitive tradition share this view of pathology and disease, often working closely with clinicians in the interests of enhancing their ability to treat and prevent diseases. As I now go on to discuss, the biographical approach to genetic diseases shares some of these reductionist foundations, although it also moves beyond the psychosocial approach in other important respects.

Biography narratives

Research into families' experiences of living with a child affected by a genetic disorder has moved from the psychosocial approach which focused upon the burden of the child, to a more nuanced approach which looks at the child's integration within the family. This often involves narratives about the family and their shared histories; themes of coping, normalization and adaptation are also present. It is argued, for example, that families cope well with rearing disabled children, and although their difficulties may be magnified when a child in need of care is present, their experiences are not dissimilar from families without a disabled child (Pelchart *et al.*, 2003). Work on parents' experiences of perceived stigma also counters the focus of much of the earlier work on the so-called objective burden of the disease (although, as we shall see, this has not entirely disappeared from the analysis) (Green, 2003). Other works suggest that families embrace, rather than reject, the paradox of loving their disabled child as they are, and wishing that their disability could be avoided, and constructing narratives of hope for the future (Larson, 1998). Unfortunately, most of the work on the experience of disability in families does not involve interviews with children so it is difficult to know how they give narrative form to their own lives and those of their carers (Mulderij, 1996, is an exception).

A large proportion of qualitative research into the experiences of families affected by genetic diseases concerns their uptake of genetics tests and the factors that influence this process. This work emphasizes the dynamics of the family, and how this shapes their response to the test. Similar work on people's experiences of managing genetic risk also considers their coping strategies in the context of family life. Much of this recent work focuses upon biographical narratives as a way of understanding people's experiences. I now turn to consider three examples of research in this genre, to assess the extent to which it reflects the biomedical model that also shaped the psychosocial model of research into patients' perspectives.

Shepherd and colleagues from the Department of Diabetes and Vascular Medicine at the University of Exeter conducted a study entitled 'Predictive Genetic Testing in Diabetes: A Case Study of Multiple Perspectives' in 2000. Their study focused upon the biographical experiences and motivations for testing as discussed by members of one at-risk family, the competing priorities in genetic counselling, and the different attitudes to predictive testing for children among family members and health professionals. The father has a hereditary form of diabetes and his daughter was contemplating predictive testing to see if she might also be affected. Shepherd and colleagues suggest that the father and daughter had engaged in a process of normalization, as they coped with the impact of the condition upon the family. They noted that the father experienced aspects of a spoilt identity and loss of self, and expressed resentment about his illness. They also noted that his attitudes shifted in the course of the interviews, as he reflected on his past. This was presented as evidence that as chronic illness unfolds over the life course, peoples' perspectives on it change. The authors note that predictive testing was popular with this family because they thought it would reduce their uncertainty. Their paper has its own narrative, noting towards the end that the family were 'empowered' by the results of the test. The authors go on to summarize their results, and those of similar studies:

> The autobiographical experience of diabetes was a key factor influencing the motivation for testing in this particular family and it has been previously described as a strong motivation in other diseases... In conjunction with other studies into managing life with a chronic condition in which a system of normalization emerged... our findings also reveal how this family with diabetes normalized aspect of their daily lives... and constructed a story of life with a chronic disease as normal.
>
> (ibid.: 256)

They conclude that their finding, among others, will help counsellors trying to explore their clients' misconceptions about genetics and inheritance, enabling them to tailor information to suit their needs.

This paper emphasizes the families' strategies of normalization and coping, and their transition from uncertainty to relief because of the test. Their biography explained their decision to take the test. The test result became part of the families' process of normalization. For the authors it is evidence of the value of these kinds of predictive tests. The stress here is upon the benefits of genetic information in helping people to normalize. This reflects a biomedical model of disease where the father's physical pathology results in the family's psychological pathology (anxiety) that can be solved by counselling and information about their risk status. However, the family was also presented as coping with their risk through other processes of normalization that occurred out with the clinical context. Their clinical encounters were presented as complementary to these coping strategies.

This positive emphasis upon normalization and coping can also be found in other research into people's experiences of living with a genetic condition, which focus upon biography narratives. Regina Kenen, a sociologist, and Audrey Ardern-Jones and Rosalind Eeles from the Royal Marsden Hospital, have studied how healthy women with a family history of breast/ovarian cancer manage their risk (Kenen *et al.*, 2003). Their work gives important insights into the perspectives and experiences of people with family histories of genetic disease. They do not argue that widespread predictive testing for disease is a 'quick fix' to these families' predicament. However, the biomedical model of disease is implicitly reinforced in their work in other respects. The authors argue that the women in their study used various coping strategies to 'get on with their lives'. They draw parallels between these women's experiences and those of people 'suffering with chronic illness' (*sic*), including notions of biographic disruption. Women's accounts of anxiety, and ways of minimizing it are highlighted. Kenen and colleague note that this often involved the women keeping their worries to themselves, as well as making specific health and lifestyle choices designed to minimize their risks. This leads them to challenge what they represent as disability activists' stress on the positive aspects of a lifetime of disability or chronic illness, thus:

> ...the positive aspects of a chronic condition did not reflect how the women perceived their situation. What they perceived as positive were the actions they could take to reduce their increased risk.
>
> (ibid.: 327)

They conclude by calling for further research into the 'clinical usefulness of these concepts to understanding attitudes and behaviors of clients attending cancer genetics risk clinics' (ibid.: 329).

This study, like the previous one, is associated with the aim of improving clinical outcomes for this group of women. As such, it has much to commend it. However, this study does not explore these women's experiences of living with these kinds of genetic histories in great depth. The authors' predominant focus is upon their subjects' risk-reduction measures. They emphasize these women's positive steps in the face of a negative and disruptive form of risk. This implicitly supports the introduction of predictive testing in this arena, and the surgical risk-reduction measures that might follow. However, the women's responses to these highly problematic approaches to managing future diseases are not discussed (see discussion of Hallowell papers in the next section).

This narrow focus can also be seen in the analogy drawn between subjects' experiences and those of patients' 'suffering' from chronic illness. This is a rather odd analogy, given that these women are, as far as we are aware, well. A more accurate comparison could have been drawn between the experiences of these women and people affected by a genetic disorder who are currently living healthy lives. For example, people with a family history of hypercholestero-laemia or HD (e.g. Lambert and Rose, 1996; Cox and McKellin, 1999). People live with risk in a range of ways, not all of which involve measures to reduce their risk. Coping is but one aspect of how people deal with a family history of genetic disease. Thinking of this as a matter of risk is by no means inevitable, or indeed helpful for many families. As Cox and McKellin, drawing on Parsons and Atkinson (1992), have previously argued, 'the relevancy of risk is...fluid and contingent: information about risk is, at certain critical junctures, given a high degree of relevance while at other times it has much less importance' (Cox and McKellin, 1999: 628). Yet, when health professionals and sociologists foreground coping with risk, they implicitly support the biomedical model of disease, and tend not to question the relevancy and value of predictive testing and risk-reduction measures in the wider context of people's lives.

The focus upon coping with one's biology is also reflected in research into the experiences of adults living with genetic disease. A recent paper by two sociologists, Karen Lowton and Jonathan Gabe, based on a project funded, in part, by Harefield NHS Trust, looked at the perceptions of health in adults with CF (Lowton and Gabe, 2003). This is an important study in an under-researched area. Health professionals often make assumptions about what it is like to live with a genetic disease, but there is not much solid empirical research to support these assumptions. As Lowton and Gabe argue, CF is typically seen as a disease of childhood, and adults' experiences of the disease are often ignored.

Lowton and Gabe concentrate upon their subjects' styles and ways of coping with the disease in relation to several processes of biographical disruption. They identify what they call four stages of disease – health as normal, health as controllable, health as distressing and health as a release, noting that:

> these concepts can be viewed as cyclical, with movement around the cycle being influenced by stage of disease, form of treatment and social context .... Two styles for maintaining these health perceptions were identified .... These were fraudulence in claims to be seen as an adult with CF and denial of the disease or its effects. Three specific modes of coping and associated strategies were also identified. These were comparisons with others, seen either as healthy or with CF; maintenance of a positive attitude; and acknowledgement and minimizing loss of spontaneity.
>
> (Lowton and Gabe, 2003: 314)

Their analysis emphasizes the complexity and variability of people's experiences, noting positive aspects of people's experiences and ways of coping, and reflecting upon their experiences in relation to other people's experiences of health and illness. However, the emphasis upon fraudulence and denial are less sympathetic. The authors still place considerable emphasis upon the biological circumstances that shape peoples' coping strategies. When the two do not tally in their eyes, their subjects' perceptions are interpreted as forms of self-deception or denial, suggesting that they are experiencing psychological as well as biological deficiencies. The biological factors influencing their perceptions are also foregrounded in the following quote:

> Death is not mentioned, but it would be an obvious alternative pathway from health as a distressing state. Indeed, much of the uncertainty and variability found in CF patients' perceptions of health arises from the fact that 'there is still no evidence of a particular age being a crisis point at which mortality rises sharply' (Dodge *et al*. 496). Adults can die at any time...
>
> (Lowton and Gabe, 2003: 315)

Here the authors seem to be suggesting that when CF adult's concepts of health vary it is partly because they cannot cope with uncertainty about when they will die. This implies that shortcomings in their ability to rationalize their situation are the result of their fatal biomedical condition. Looked at from another perspective, it could be argued that all of us have varying perceptions of our health, and the fact that most of us do not know when we will die does not mean we are necessarily psychologically disturbed. Lack of knowledge about when we will die could even be interpreted as a reason for some people's positive outlook on life. Adults with CF may share some of these perspectives too, despite their illness.

When sociologists highlight the biological roots of perception they take attention away from the social contexts in which illnesses are experienced and understood. Feelings of desperation or hope can be engendered by a range of human relationships. They are not always rooted in the physical state of one's body. Variations in one's perceptions of health do not necessarily signal denial or inability to cope with death, but result from a whole range of social relations. People can hold quite contradictory perceptions of health and disease simultaneously. Too much of a focus upon people's ability to cope with their current or future biological processes takes attention away from this complexity and tends to support the biomedical approach to identifying and treating diseases as early and as aggressively as possible.

The context of the interviews on which these types of studies are based also requires more careful consideration. When people are asked to talk about their experiences of illness, by people associated with the hospital where they are treated, their clinical experiences shape their accounts. Discourses of wanting to know about one's risk, being ready to act to minimize it, and being able to cope with one's illness, are common within this context. People will tend to adopt the position of 'patient' in interviews with researchers, following the model that they already know from the doctor–patient encounter. As Bury has argued, asking people to talk about illness *per se* provokes quite specific forms of illness narrative, that are not typically focused upon the mundane aspects of their experiences (Bury, 2001; see also Lawton, 2003). If they were asked to talk generally about genetics, not their illness, by people outside of the medical setting, one might get a very different narrative about their experiences of their condition in relation to employment, campaigning or charity work, their views on research into gene therapy and so on. This might involve discussion of how they experienced their bodies and how they accounted for periods of illness or anxiety about future illness, but the wider social context of which these experiences were a part would be much more apparent.

Risk and responsibility

I now turn to consider some studies of people's experiences of genetic diseases that move beyond individuals' illness narratives and a focus upon coping, to explore experience in a wider context. I am interested in the extent to which these studies challenge, or reinforce the predominant themes in patient research – normalization and the biological conditions which shape them.

Nina Hallowell has conducted a considerable amount of research into the experiences of women attending genetic counselling for hereditary breast and ovarian cancer. She has also analysed women's accounts of their perception of risk and the positive steps they might take to reduce that risk. However, Hallowell takes a broader, more contextual approach than some other studies, analysing women's perceptions of responsibility to their family and the importance of putting others' needs before their own (Hallowell, 1999). She finds that this meant that they

> Justified their willingness to adopt potentially harmful risk management practices as motivated by their obligations to fulfill others' needs: to engage in mothering work, to prevent family members from seeing them suffering or having to care for them and to provide dying relatives with peace of mind. Thus, it can be argued, that these women's risk management choices are constrained by those gendered discourses which position women as responsible for the care of others, for they regard their ability to fulfill their obligations of care as dependent upon them taking steps to control their risk.
>
> (ibid.: 612–13)

Although Hallowell goes on to note that this does not necessarily mean that these choices are disempowering, they are far from a matter of autonomous agents making rational decisions about reducing their objective genetic risks. The choices and the risks they concern are profoundly moral.

In a later paper, written with Julia Lawton, Hallowell develops this analysis, to argue that risk-reduction measures are not necessarily a means of control, or normalization, as is suggested in other works. Focusing upon prophylactic surgery, they note that this can be associated with a sense of loss of control. This, they argue, means that 'women's willingness to undergo prophylactic ovarian surgery is dependent upon them negotiating various competing risks to self and body that are associated with this risk management option' (Hallowell and Lawton, 2002: 423). In this analysis, cancer patient becomes one of a number of anticipated biographies, as does older woman (surgery brings on early menopause). They also note that surgically induced menopause was not perceived as a chronic illness, but that the after-effects of surgery were viewed as biographically disruptive.

These studies present a much more sophisticated analysis of people's experiences of genetic risk than much of the work in the biographical narrative genre. The biological conditions or potential biological conditions at stake are not treated as if they were the main factor shaping women's perceptions of their risk or health, instead they are presented as one part of a wider complex of familial relationships and self-identities. The benefits of presymptomatic testing, and the prophylactic risk-reduction measures with which they are associated, are questions, not simply assumed, by participants and analysts alike. Coping takes various forms. Normalization is resisted in some cases, just as it is embraced in others. This is not a matter of the research subjects being engaged in self-deception or denial, but of them managing the risks and responsibilities of their lives in relation to their bodies and the social (and technical) networks of which they are a part.

Hallowell's work is nevertheless part of the genre of clinic-based studies that dominate this field. As such, it gives a partial perspective on women's experiences of hereditary risk in the context of their daily lives. Other more anthropologically focused work has, however, moved out of the clinic, to the community as a whole. How are risk and responsibility contextualized in these types of study?

Kaja Finkler has conducted research into the ways in which people made sense of family and kinship relations when new genetic information about their risk status comes to light. Finkler and colleagues have argued that 'family and kinship relations are being medicalized as a result of the current emphasis on medical genetics and its clinical applications' (Finkler *et al.*, 2003: 403). They continue:

> in mainstream American society, emphasis is laid on biogenetic kinship, which defines families by the sharing of genes, removes the possibility of choosing one's relatives.... While people may select who they will love [with some exceptions] among those in their biogenetic group, biomedicine insists on uniting those who may not feel connected or who may not choose to be united ... the medicalization of family and kinship provided empirical proof to the layman that the disease is genetic because they

witness other family members experiencing the same or similar affliction
.... People do consider other explanations, especially environmental factors . . . but these explanations are more often than not discarded in favour
of the prevailing genetic explanation.

(ibid.: 406)

Finkler and colleagues present the case of 'Dorothy' to support their
argument. Dorothy's mother and maternal grandmother died of breast cancer, and she is fearful that she will also develop the disease. She has yearly
mammographies but has decided against predictive genetic testing because
she does not think it would be '100 per cent definite'. The authors argue:

> This profound concern diminishes her daily existence by leaving her in a
> state of unceasing doubt and fear about her risk.... At the same time, she
> embraces a sense of fatalism that sanctioned her becoming a mother. The
> unwavering belief in genetic inheritance has, however, brought her closer
> to her blood kin, and motivated her to learn more about her family history.
>
> (ibid.: 407)

For Finkler and colleagues, Dorothy has already become a patient, and like many
others lives with a 'fear of the future', 'clamour[ing] for an illusory certainty that
they desire from testing' (ibid.: 408). In this way, people 'can even find meaning
in the randomness of an affliction' (ibid.), as they establish connections with
family members that have been lost. This, however, means that the individual is
no longer the sole patient – the family becomes the central focus.

Throughout this chapter, I have been arguing that health professionals and
their allies in the social sciences have, to some extent, created and extended
the category of patient through the research that is conducted into their experiences. I have suggested that this means that we have lost sight of the different identities of people affected by genetic disease; and that we have
exaggerated the place of genetic risk or impairment in their lives. I have suggested that these studies biologize people's experiences of genetic disease,
rooting them in biological risks rather than the social conditions of their
lives. The extent to which patients are coping; their levels of anxiety; their
ability to rationalize – all of these qualities are treated as if they were in some
ways determined by their biological functions – the symptoms and severity
of their impairment.

Finkler and colleagues appear to be engaged in the same types of biolo-
gization of experience in order to support their argument about the medicalization of family and kinship. Their analysis of people's sense of risks and
responsibilities are as narrow as those of the clinicians they criticize. At a time
when many social scientists are looking to the complexities of people's identities and experiences, Finkler and colleagues choose to focus on those features
of contemporary life that support their argument. Their discussion of

medicalization does not take account of the fluidity of family relationships and practices of intimacy in contemporary societies, including America, or the range of different discourses about the causes of health and disease that people draw on when discussing these matters. They identify new trends and attribute these to biomedical developments. For example, a growing interest in genealogy is linked to developments in medical genetics. They suggest that people now tend to attribute illness to heredity factors rather than the environment. This, too, is a result of developments in genetics. However, the empirical evidence for all of these claims is slight.

Dorothy, interviewed by Finkler, is apparently consumed with fear and driven by a search for certainty: an inevitable patient. However, Dorothy has presented a particular narrative to Finkler, and Finkler has focused upon the aspects of her account that suggested medicalization. Dorothy's rejection of the genetic test could be interpreted as ambivalence about her status as a patient, as could her choice to have children, choices which are, after all, being discussed here retrospectively in the context of an interview about one aspect of what is I am sure a full and complex life. Leaving aside these doubts, it is difficult to accept Finkler and colleagues' claim that Dorothy represents most of the American women facing these types of situation. Other evidence from studies of women affected by genetic disease in their families, such as the work by Hallowell discussed earlier, does not present such a grim tale of inevitable patients. Although their choices were obviously shaped by concerns for family, they were far from inevitable.

There is a very real danger that when genetic risk is foregrounded in research studies, its impact and importance in people's lives can be exaggerated. In the same way as health professionals who are supportive of genetic testing can emphasize quite narrow aspects of patients' experiences, researchers who are critical of genetic testing can do the same. Participants can also tend to position themselves as patients in an effort to be helpful to people who are interviewing them. This might mean that they selectively discuss various aspects of their experiences of family and kinship that they can relate to their genetic risk, and in so doing give the impression that these aspects of their relationships are more fundamental or important than they might be if they were discussed in another context. They may also imply causal links, and construct chains of events which place the genetic diagnosis or risk on centre-stage, implying that changing relationships have resulted from this one event, presenting a rather determinist version of family life. This is not to say that genetic diagnoses do not impact upon individuals and families in these ways, just that they are part of a much broader picture, subject to change and reinterpretation, which means that their significance should not be overplayed.

Novas and Rose's work on debates among those at risk of developing HD and their relatives, gives an insight into some of these complexities, and warns against the type of analysis advanced by Finkler and colleagues, and others critical of the new genetics, on the basis that it medicalizes or geneticizes people's experiences. Crucially, they argue:

> Genetic risks does not imply resignation in the face of an implacable biological destiny: it induces new and active relations to oneself and one's future... the mutations in personhood associated with the new life sciences and bio-medical technologies of life are multiple and not simply genetic... Ideas about biological, biomedical and genetic identity will certainly infuse, interact, combine and contest with other identity claims; we doubt they will supplant them.
>
> (Novas and Rose, 2000: 485)

This takes us well beyond the domain of the patient in genetic research, to the ways in which people affected by genetic disorders maintain a range of different positions in relation to their disease, and engage in a range of relationships with members of their family. Although Novas and Rose do not present much empirical data to support their case, other work in this field also shows that people do not simply accept genetic diagnoses. Nor do they always want to know their risk status. If they prefer to remain ignorant, it is not necessarily because they are deluded or deranged, but because this strategy makes sense in their lives at that particular time (Cox and McKellin, 1999). Genetic diagnoses can reshape family relationships, but this is not inevitable, nor is this simply a one-way process. Family relationships also shape people's attitude to taking the test in the first place. Experiencing a genetic disorder, as an affected individual, or a family member, involves much more than taking a test or engaging in risk-prevention. People affected in these ways can become experts in their own right, or campaigners and activists. They may feel that they are constrained by others who cannot conceive of them as anything other than patients, but there are ways in which these roles can be subverted and resisted, via support groups and web-based networks, for example (see Stockdale, 1999). As Lawton notes with respect to the work of Ville and colleagues (1994), it is important to locate 'illness experiences in "collective" contexts', such as the disability movement, where positive images of disability also shape people's self-identities and their capacity to interpret their experiences in different ways (Lawton, 2003, drawing on Ville *et al.*, 1994).

Other work on families' experiences of caring for a disabled child also emphasizes the importance of culture and traditions to the ways in which familial responsibilities are enacted. Anderton and colleagues studied the different approaches of Chinese and white families to physiotherapy and the use of prosthetics (Anderton *et al.*, 1989). They noted that Chinese families found it difficult to find the resources to engage in these activities, but that they also encouraged their child to take them up so that they could be fit for work. White families were more concerned with aesthetic normality. This sets the processes of 'normalization' within a much richer frame of family and community life, which allows us to see normalization as a kind of ideology, rather than a simple social fact. However, as Lawton and others, such as Atkin and colleagues (1998) have argued: 'we should not push the medical context too far to the sidelines' (Lawton, 2003: 32). Problems with access to services and resources fundamentally shape people's experiences of illness. When families are from minority ethnic communities, these problems can be especially galling. As Atkin and colleagues point out: 'racialized stereotypes and the inability to meet the linguistic and cultural needs of affected groups' (Atkin *et al.*, 1998: 51), mean that some children in minority families affected by haemoglobinopathies are being denied the position of patient, and dying needlessly as a result.

Looking directly to the accounts of people affected by genetic disorders can also help to illuminate the various identities which they assume and how their bodies and relationships with other people shape these identities (see Morris, 1996; Shakespeare *et al.*, 1996; Thomas, 1999). Despite a long-standing interest in the disability community in telling their own stories, it is difficult to find many first-hand accounts of people's experiences of genetic disorders. Several accounts are presented in Teresa Marteau and Martin Richard's edited collection *The Troubled Helix* (1996) and in Eric Parens and Adrienne Asch's *Prenatal Testing and Disability Rights* (2000). These personal narratives are written for different reasons, for different audiences. *The Troubled Helix* has a short précis that captures its approach well:

> The availability of increasingly sophisticated information on our genetic make-up presents individuals and society as a whole, with difficult decisions. Although it is hoped that these advances will ultimately lead the way to the effective treatment and screening for all diseases with a genetic component, at present many individuals as 'condemned' to a life sentence in the knowledge that they, or their children, will suffer from an incurable genetic disease.
>
> (Marteau and Richards, 1996)

Parens and Asch's book is based on a dialogue between people in the disability rights community and health professionals and scholars, so the book is described on the cover as setting out to 'debate the implications of prenatal testing for people with disabilities and for parent–child relationships generally'. This leads to quite different first-hand narratives.

Marteau and Richards present stories from people affected by four types of genetic conditions – HD, hereditary breast and ovarian cancer, Werdnig-Hoffman's syndrome and Sickle-cell conditions. A total of eleven stories are presented, with introductions to each disease section by the editors, and a final section with the reactions of a clinical geneticist. The people who provided these accounts are described by the editors as 'living in the shadow of genetic disease' (ibid.: xv). They were asked only to write about their personal experience. The editors express the hope that they will 'remind readers not only of the pain and misery that genetic disorders can cause and the dilemmas that they may pose for family members, but also the very varied ways in which people choose to live their lives in the face of an inherited condition' (ibid.: 4). Of the three accounts of living with HD, two of the authors chose to undergo genetic testing, and one has yet to decide. The editors acknowledge that this is not a representative sample of people with a family history of HD, noting that only a small minority chose to undergo testing.

This presentation of people's first-hand experiences of genetic disease is clearly shaped by a biomedical model of disease, and a focus upon how people negotiate knowledge about risk. These accounts nevertheless present a complex picture of what it means to be at risk of a genetic disease, as the authors reflect upon the stigma and discrimination they have experienced, their responsibilities to their families and unborn children, the benefits and drawbacks of counselling and their relationships with friends. They also give insights into other aspects of their lives, which are in the words of one author, 'nothing to do with HD', but affect their relationships nonetheless. Their ambivalence about predictive genetic test results is palpable, but the extent to which they were concerned about risk varied considerably, depending upon their situations, as the following extract illustrates:

> On the whole my life continues to be fully occupied – with children and work, not to mention worries about a failing business and new job – for worries about Huntington's disease to hold sway. Nevertheless, since the birth of my daughter I have noticed a change in my attitude to being at risk of the disease, with a considerable increase both in the extent to which it preoccupies and concerns me, and in the extent to which I look out for and find possible symptoms in myself. One reason for this is that although my father's symptoms are still far from overwhelming, they have become more marked recently. In addition, some shift has taken place in my mind with the certainty that my child-bearing days are now over, which to me implies no longer being 'young'. I have reached a point where I must acknowledge that Huntington's disease commonly manifests itself in people of my age.
> (Anonymous, in Marteau and Richards, 1996: 24)

This quote illustrates how people's accounts of genetic risk are relative to their sense of connections to family members, their role in the workforce, as well as the physical state of their bodies and those of other people's bodies.

In the accounts of people affected by Werdnig-Hoffman's syndrome, genetic risk is presented as coming to the fore with the decision to take a prenatal test: a decision that is often based on the experience of already having a child who died at an early age as a result of the condition. This is an altogether different form of risk from that of HD or hereditary breast cancer. Parents face the risk of Werdnig-Hoffman's syndrome at quite specific points in pregnancy, often after the very distressing experience of a child's death. Even so, the accounts in this volume suggest that this form of genetic risk is not necessarily always at the forefront of parents' minds. Parents' relationships with families and social support networks as well as health professionals as also presented as having shaped their perceptions of genetic risk.

The accounts presented in Parens and Asch's volume are shorter and more specifically focused upon the issue of prenatal testing. One in particular stands out because it is the perspective of a woman who is largely at ease with her genetic disorder – a form of hereditary blindness. Deborah Kent writes:

> I premised my life on the conviction that blindness was a neutral charac-teristic. It created some inconveniences, such as not being able to read print or drive a car. Occasionally, it locked me into conflicts with others over what I could and could not do. But in the long run I believed that my life had not always turned out any better if I had been fully sighted. If my child were blind, I would try to ensure it every chance to become a self-fulfilled contributing member of society.
>
> (Kent in Parens and Asch, 2000: 58)

Kent goes on to discuss how her husband and her parents negotiated their differences when her daughter was born (sighted). This illustrates some of the ways in which genetic risks are negotiated by family members, and translated in the light of their new experiences.

Conclusion

There are still many gaps in analyses of people's experiences of genetic diseases. These remain focused upon the experiences of a relatively affluent and articulate minority of adults affected by late-onset genetic disorders, the work of Rapp and Atkin and others notwithstanding. Children's accounts of their experiences of genetic disorders are almost entirely absent from this lit-erature. There is a lack of attention to the experiences of families from minor-ity ethnic communities, and disabled people who reject genetic technologies, such as prenatal testing. Alongside these serious omissions, there is another set of seemingly less important gaps in our knowledge of the more mundane aspects of living with genetic disorders. Much of this work focuses upon peo-ple's attitudes to genetic diagnosis and its ramifications, not the place of genetics in their daily lives. However, I would argue that these stories of ordi-nary life are an important antidote to the tendency to focus upon the partic-ularities of the clinical context and the accounts of risk and responsibility that reflection about this can generate. Genetic risk is not ever present. It forms part of people's life worlds, without necessarily dominating them at all times. People do not always want to minimize or cope with genetic risk – sometimes they want to ignore it and at other times to foreground it. Sometimes people want to be patients, at other times they do not. People can also be different types of patients – informed, ignorant, active, passive, independent, depend-ent. These roles and the discourses they are associated with, depend upon people's social location and context. They are shaped by their experiences of their impairments, but also by their experiences of relationships with health care providers, family members, friends, colleagues, members of their communities and even researchers. People's interpretation of genetic risk and their decision to take a test and to act on the results, are also shaped by these social relations. However, people are not patients, most of the time, they are mothers, sisters, professionals, schoolchildren, friends, customers and much more. Focusing upon 'patients' experiences beyond the clinic gives but a partial perspective on the ways in which people live with genetic disorders.

Further reading

Bury, M. (2001) 'Illness narratives: facts or fiction?', *Sociology of Health and Illness*, 23:3, 263–85.

Cox, S. and McKellin, W. (1999) 'There's this thing in our family: predictive testing and the construction of risk for Huntington's Disease', *Sociology of Health and Illness*, 21:5, 622–46.

Hallowell, N. and Lawton, J. (2002) 'Negotiating present and future selves: managing the risk of hereditary ovarian cancer by prophylactic surgery', *Health*, 6:4, 423–43.

Lawton, J. (2003) 'Lay experiences of health and illness: past research and future agendas', *Sociology of Health and Illness*, 25:3, 23–40.

6 Biobanks

Summary

This chapter explores the governance of genetic research through the case of biobanking. Biobanks involve considerable negotiation over the collection, storage and acceptable use of DNA, which involves setting up and enacting specific protocols of informed consent and confidentiality. This chapter explores the ways in which these protocols are presented in the professional literature, and the discourses of informed consent and social progress that this involves. I also explore what happens when donation occurs, and the ways in which information and consent are negotiated in the process. I am especially interested in how tensions about the rights and responsibilities of the different actors involved in biobanking are negotiated in the clinic and beyond in the public sphere.

I go on to consider how research subjects are variously constructed as patients by proxy and active health consumers, in professional discussions about informed consent and confidentiality. However, biobanks are also highly public ventures. This has meant that a range of competing subject positions also exist alongside that of patient and health consumer, particularly the position of citizen. I consider the ways in which doctors and scientists involved with biobanks negotiate these different positions, which involves considerable reflexivity about their own status as ethical professionals.

Introduction

So far, we have been considering genetic technologies that are used in the diagnosis or treatment of individuals affected by genetic disease or defined populations such as pregnant women or people with hereditary forms of cancer. We have also been exploring the ways in which genetic discoveries occur, mainly focusing upon the identification of genes involved in rare and serious genetic diseases such as cystic fibrosis. We have explored the various ways in which appeals to individual choice, scientific progress and the treatment of disease are represented by advocates and critics alike.

In this chapter, we consider these discourses in relation to another area of genetic research – genetic databanks, or biobanks as they will be called here.

GeneWatch UK estimates that there may already be as many as 300 biobanks in the United Kingdom in the field of cancer research alone. These collections are typically small, but bigger population-based databanks, which combine a range of medical, genealogical and genetic information have also been established. The pharmaceutical industry and biotechnology sector has established collections, some of which are based on samples routinely collected during clinical trials, but others, such as that held by Oxagen, are based on samples from families with specific diseases, such as coronary artery disease. These biobanks tend not to be subject to the same level of ethical scrutiny as ones in the public sector. One of the largest public UK biobanks is held by the Avon Longitudinal Study of Parents and Children (ALSPAC), which has data from 14,000 families from the Avon area who have been monitored since 1991. The UK Biobank, for which collections are due to begin in 2004, is on an altogether larger scale, with plans for an estimated 500,000 samples to be collected over a seven-year period. This mirrors the situation internationally, where at least half-a-dozen countries as well as some US health providers have established biobanks.

These biobanks hold information on a large number of people, many of whom are not directly affected by genetic disease, *per se*. This extends public involvement with genetic research to a far greater number of people than ever before. A large amount of medical, lifestyle and genetic information is being stored in these databases, raising many concerns about privacy and confidentiality in the so-called information society. These biobanks are designed to aid research into common diseases in the rich West – cancer, heart disease and stroke. Increasingly biobanks take the form of public–private partnerships, given their considerable commercial potential in terms of drug development. One of the most controversial ventures of this sort is that of the Icelandic government and deCode Genetics – the Icelandic Health Sector Database, which combines the health records and genetic information of the Icelandic population.

Biobanks are popular because it is hoped that they will enable scientists to identify the involvement of genes in a range of complex diseases, thereby leading to better treatments and prevention plans. They are surrounded by a discourse of promise and discovery, but are not without controversy, particularly around issues of the informed consent of donors. The Icelandic Health Sector Database has been heavily criticized by the international community and the Icelandic Medical Association because of its presumed consent policy, which runs counter to the standard model of informed consent for DNA donation for medical research. This database also raises questions about the synergy between government and private capital. DeCode claimed to be acting in the interests of the Icelandic economy, but it is currently making a loss, and this has affected many ordinary Icelanders with shares in the company (Meek, 2002).

Researchers hold different views on the best way in which to organize such biobanks on scientific as well as ethical grounds. They dispute the optimum characteristics of the cohort and the quality of the health information provided to biobanks. Promises of benefits such as personalized health plans and treatments have also been questioned. UK Biobank has attracted controversy because of the large sums of money that are being spent (estimates vary from £40 to £60 million) on what some see as a grand vision which lacks rigorous and open governance structures and clear scientific hypotheses (Barbour, 2003). Although public consultation has taken place, and people expressed concerns about the potential for the proposed collection to lead to discrimination, biobank's managers have not specifically addressed them. This has increased concern about the extent to which the public's views will shape the governance of UK Biobank (Kerr, 2003).

In this chapter, I will consider the ways in which the rights and responsibilities of patients, professionals and other so-called stakeholders such as the community or government are represented in the professional literature and reports about biobanks. I will explore the way that notions of social good and progress are used as arguments in support of biobanks, and the arguments against them. Other discussions about risk will also be considered. These are divided into three substantive areas. The first concerns the collection, storage and initial use of DNA in biobanks, covering important issues such as informed consent, confidentiality, and communication of results to donors and their families. This section also considers the ways in which some other potential uses of the information stored in medical genetic databanks, for example, by pharmaceutical companies, are presented, and how this is related to the issue of informed consent. Two other areas to be addressed are the issues of ownership and governance of this type of biomedical research. I will address the patenting discussion, but also distribution of benefits more generally, alongside the framing of governance roles of professionals, donors and the community at large. Throughout I will try to deconstruct the discourses around these aspects of biobanks, and introduce some sociological and anthropological work on participants' perspectives to illuminate the practices that they involve.

In the past, many clinicians routinely retained tissue samples from their patients for future research. However, recent high profile scandals about the retention without permission of children's organs at the Bristol Royal Infirmary and the Alder Hey Hospital have dented public confidence in the medical profession, and led organizations like the General Medical Council to issue new guidelines that require explicit informed consent for retention of tissue samples. These changes occurred alongside new developments in genetic sequencing technologies and information technology. A range of organizations and individuals, from scientific, legal, ethical and medical backgrounds, expressed concerns about misuse of the information that they might generate about individual's susceptibility to disease. Other broader developments such as increasing links between the biotechnology industry and academia, and various high profile controversies about patenting life, have intensified discussion in the public domain about the exploitation of medical information for commercial benefit. The growth of institutional bioethics in the form of ethics committees, and national and international committees and working parties have also put the ethics of genetic research under the spotlight (Kerr and Shakespeare, 2002).

These developments have all shaped the ways in which the ethics of biobanks are framed by their advocates and critics alike. Researchers and organizers tend to favour the establishment of new databases as opposed to the use of old sample collections, and they place the issue of informed consent on centre-stage, as do their critics. This separates their work from the past, orienting it in the imagined future of individualized health care and focusing upon donors' rights. Organizers and overseers of these new biobanks focus in particular upon donors' rights to privacy and confidentiality, reflecting the current emphasis upon individual choice in much of biomedicine. Genetic information tends to be presented as having a special status, because of what it can reveal about the health of a person's relatives or future generations. This makes the issue of how and when results are communicated to donors and their relatives particularly important in the governance of biobanks. These issues will now be addressed in turn.

Informed consent

The Icelandic Health Sector Database has been heavily criticized by researchers, social scientists, ethicists and privacy-campaigners the world over, because of the system of 'presumed consent' on which it is based. Icelandic scientists and clinicians, alongside their international counterparts, have criticized the database, because in the words of one critic, it is a 'serious breach of ethics in medical research' (McInnis, 1999: 234). Informed consent is frequently described as 'a cornerstone of the ethics of medical research' (ibid.: 235), developed in response to the barbarism of Nazi medicine. Data protection and human rights legislation have further underlined the importance of individuals' rights to informed consent to participate in research that will gather and store information about them. The protocols of a range of national and international agencies concerned with biomedical ethics echo these themes. The principle of informed consent has come to underline physicians' responsibilities to explain research, including its risks, to their patients. Many doctors would argue that if they did not seek informed consent for this kind of research, their patients would lose trust in them and biomedical researchers share this interest in informed consent. In the words of one multidisciplinary group charged with developing an informed consent form for population genetic studies:

> Society currently invests an enormous power in the concept of genetics, and, considering the history of eugenics and other research abuses ... [so] clarifying the obligations of investigators to participants in population-based research involving genetics is important.
>
> (Beskow *et al.*, 2001: 2316)

An emphasis upon informed consent is one means by which researchers can signal that their practices are ethical, and show that they are able to address what they view as a crisis of public trust about their expertise and intentions. Informed consent also speaks to the increasing emphasis upon individuals' rights, which reflects the growing culture of consumerism in health care. This reflects other more bureaucratic and litigious conditions too. Rigorous standards of informed consent in biomedical research protect institutions, as well as patients. Typically, informed consent forms for DNA banking involve a statement which informs donors that the researchers' institution may patent discoveries made with their DNA sample, and that they will not receive any royalties. Informed consent forms limit donor's rights of ownership. They also give donors' responsibility, for considering the consequences of the research. Critics such as Merz and colleagues have argued that this assumes that the 'subjects act solely because of altruism and that the sole duty of researchers is to disclose their intentions' (Merz *et al.*, 2002: 965), thus reducing the complex interplay of social and cultural conditions which shape the process of donation.

Helen Busby conducted interviews with donors to genetic research into the causes of psoriatic arthritis, a disease that affects skin and joints. She found that the process of giving informed consent was highly ambiguous, particularly when participants seemed to pay little heed to the genetic aspect of the study, assuming that it was 'good modern science' and that DNA was nothing special, except in the sense that it was linked with expectations of cures and treatments resulting from the research. Their consent was also bound up with a sense of confidence in the NHS and the university sector (Busby, 2004). Others have shown that patient groups play an important role in generating in this 'political economy of hope' (Stockdale, 1999). Klaus Hoeyer echoes these findings, stressing that people involved in the Swedish biobank he has been studying have a range of relationships with the blood that they donate and the information to which it can be linked. Yet, the company constructs the ethical domain around blood donation rather than lifestyle or health information. Ethics becomes more or less synonymous with informed consent. Once the blood is transformed into information, it can be patented and sold without ethical discussion. Concerns about commodification become muted in favour of discussions about confidentiality and privacy, shifting the discourse from ethics to law. This denies the complexity of people's sense of where personhood resides, in genetic material and personal information (Hoeyer, 2002). In a later piece, Hoeyer also explores the work that signing an informed consent form does for participants, placing it within a much wider discussion of responsibility than is traditionally the case. This leads him to suggest that the act of signing an informed consent form is a way in which individuals can present themselves as responsible subjects, rather than as responsible for the research outcomes. This must be understood in relation to the Swedish context, where there is a strong sense of public trust in the state, particularly in northern Sweden where the research is taking place.

He suggests that this might mean that donors actively maintain the security of trust in the health care provider, and do not raise the issue of what happens to their sample in order to preserve this. He speculates that trust in the system breaks down when they are interviewed by him because he asks questions which require them to reconnect the sample to their sense of personhood (Hoeyer, 2004).

The relationship between researchers and research subjects is clearly more complex than the standard informed consent model suggests. Its role within the research context is far from unambiguous. As McQueen has argued, there is a lack of consensus among researchers and ethics committees about what kind of information ought to be provided to subjects, at what point and in what form (McQueen, 1998). This ambiguity about researchers' responsibilities is often expressed in terms of what it is reasonable for participants to expect to be told about the research, with some arguing that participants are being given too little information on which to make a decision, and others arguing that they are being over informed and cannot process large amounts of complex information (Lyttle, 1997).

Researchers and ethics committees can also have widely different interpretations of the types of consent that ought to be sought from research participants. Some researchers and institutions favour 'blanket consent', whereby they take on responsibilities for ethical research, and donor's rights to intervene are limited. Blanket consent is favoured on the basis that the research is open-ended, and its direction or indeed its implications cannot be predicted in advance. However, ethics committees often emphasize donor's rights to decide about the reuse of their sample, should research take a new direction (Berg, 2001), resulting in tension around biobank consent procedures.

One solution suggested by some North American lawyers and ethicists to these questions of choice would be to offer participants a menu of possible choices, allowing them to authorize only certain kinds of research (Rothstein, 2002). This authorization model could also involve patients exercising control over future uses of their genetic material (Caulfield *et al.*, 2003). Greely (1999) and Caulfield and colleagues (2003) have argued, blanket consent, covering all future forms of medical research, does not have much legal weight because it is far too general and far from true consent. In contrast, an authorization model would involve patients giving or withholding permission for particular types of research as well as 'unforeseen' research. They would be able to specify whether and in what circumstances they would wish to be re-contacted by researchers and withdraw their sample. They would also be able to set limits on the length of time the sample could be kept. This does not remove the possibility of blanket consent, but places it as one choice among a range of more restrictive options. This type of consumer choice arrangement would individualize decision-making to a high degree and demand the involvement of a range of lawyers and ethicists in advising individuals on their decision-making and seeing that their wishes were being followed. Researchers are unlikely to favour such a strong interpretation of donors' rights, given that it would interfere with their jurisdictional control over donors' participation in their research.

These matters are complicated by the issue of community consent, particularly in the United States, where concerns about the potential for discrimination or stigmatization of particular populations arising from genetic research have lead to recommendations from the US National Bioethics Advisory Commission that researchers ought to discuss group harm in the informed consent process. This raises many questions about how 'group' or 'community' are defined, and future risks are anticipated (see Sharp and Foster, 2002 and Box 6.1: Insurance and employment). Some critics have argued that there is a danger that defining communities to be consulted, in terms of ethnicity or race, will reify biological differences and lead to further discrimination against so-called minority groups. This is particularly problematic in areas of research that are more controversial, such as research that seeks to identify particular groups with predispositions to antisocial behaviour or psychiatric illness. Clinicians and researchers who want to retain their focus upon the individual donor have also argued that community consent is unworkable. They have pointed out that knowing the results of this type of research in advance, it is not possible to know which groups should be consulted, in this type of situation, or what risks they ought to consider (Reilly and Page, 1998).

Informed consent is clearly a flexible concept, where informed and consent can mean many different things. Informed consent can be formulated as an ideal type in such a way as to establish acceptable boundaries between professionals and donors, and between professionals when they are negotiating the governance and oversight of biobanks. General appeals to informed consent can signal one's commitment to ethical practice, and specific empirical evidence of ambiguities around informed consent can undermine certain biobanking arrangements in favour of others. Detailed and specific criteria of informed consent codify ethics in order to meet the different demands of the institution that support the research and the governing bodies that oversee it. Tensions are particularly apparent when the agency and expertise of research subjects are concerned. The responsibilities of professionals, to their patients, the research community and the public at large come under the spotlight when these issues are raised.

The flexibilities of informed consent are not surprising, given that the structure and function of biobanks is currently being negotiated by a range of parties. This involves experts from different specialisms in science, medicine, law and ethics, in addition to prospective donors, patients' organizations, public interest groups, ethics committees, charitable trusts, representatives from industry, the civil service, the media and the public at large. Biobanks are contested at a number of levels, which concern their design and utility as well as potential impacts, which means that neither the problem they are supposed to solve, and the clientele they are serving, are far from clear; nor are the technological or organizational arrangements on which they will be based. Framing and defining criteria for 'informed consent' are but one means of negotiating these parties' jurisdiction in these processes.

Two different models of research subjects are in operation here – passive, ill-informed donors and active, informed consumers. Both of these models relate to competing notions of patients' roles in biomedical research and clinical practice. On the one hand, research subjects are being cast as patients by proxy in the sense that individual patients are expected to comply with research. Through their participation they express their trust in biomedicine, but do not anticipate direct benefits from the research by way of treatments or cures for their particular complaints. They are, to a large extent, cast as dependent upon professionals to decide how much information they should be given about the research and what to do with the information and materials they donate. On the other hand, research subjects are given certain rights and responsibilities beyond those of the traditional patient, when they are expected to actively engage with the research process and to decide how the material and the information they donate should be used. This reflects a different understanding of patienthood, based upon active consumption of health information.

Box 6.1 Insurance and employment

Campaigners such as UK GeneWatch, have argued that biobanks may create problems for people with genetic disorders when they try to obtain insurance or employment. Although there are clear restrictions on third-party access to information in medical genetic databanks, there are some concerns that if government agencies become custodians of these databanks, they may access the information in the public interest. Other concerns about employers and insurers accessing personal genetic information are more applicable to clinical genetic tests than research databanks. As Reilly and Page have noted, 'the human genetics research community appears committed to sustaining a culture of strict patient confidentiality' (Reilly and Page, 1998). However, GeneWatch and others are concerned that knowledge about disease that develops as a result of biobank research may be used by employers or insurance companies to discriminate against particular groups identified as having a higher predisposition to certain diseases. GeneWatch note that there is a 'strong likelihood that genetic tests will be more widely used by employers in the future' (GeneWatch, 2001: 9), and their concerns do seem to be widely shared by members of the public. There is no UK law to prevent genetic discrimination, and there have already been instances of genetic discrimination in the United States. The Human Genetic Commission (HGC) have raised similar concerns in their report, *Inside Information* (2002), and have argued that there ought to be a law to prevent the 'non consensual or deceitful obtaining and/or analysis of personal genetic information for non-medical purposes' (Human Genetics Commission, 2002: 18), and that the government should ratify the European Convention on Human Rights and Biomedicine (1997), which prohibits discrimination on the grounds of genetic heritage. However, the HGC also suggest that employers may wish to offer genetic testing to an employee and recommend that these cases are brought to the HGC's attention so that they can, 'consider the implications' (ibid.: 12). UK insurers are currently bound by a 5-year moratorium on the use of information from genetic test results, unless there is a family history of Huntington's disease or the application is for life insurance in excess of 500,000 or critical illness income protection or long-term care insurance in excess of £300,000. However, there are reports of the insurance industry flouting this moratorium, and family histories of genetic disease already create problems for people trying to obtain insurance at reasonable rates.

Without legislation to prevent discrimination, researchers have the option of exploring 'group harms' with people who might be affected by the results of research based on medical genetic databanks. This is difficult, given that these groups or the harms they could experience might not be obvious in advance. Other options include consultation with identifiable groups, such as members of ethnic minorities and other disadvantaged groups with a common genetic heritage, and proposals that researchers obtain a kind of 'community consent' to research which might adversely affect them, should the results be used by insurance companies, for example (see Sharp and Foster, 2002). However, these proposals have been criticized for over extending the notion of community consent based on vague fears about the future, and thereby harming the progress of research (Reilly and Page, 1998). They may also increase discrimination by reasserting old notions of racial or ethnic identity (see Box 6.2).

Privacy and confidentiality

Donors' rights to consent, and to withdrawal of consent should their views change, are often stressed when the ethics of biobanks are discussed. This follows from the prevailing emphasis upon patients' rights to privacy and confidentiality, as articulated in a range of ethical pronouncements. For example, the World Medical Association's (WMA) Declaration on Ethical Considerations Regarding Health Databases, states that:

> The right to privacy entitles people to exercise control over the use and disclosure of information about them as individuals. The privacy of a patient's personal health information is secured by the physician's duty of confidentiality.... Confidentiality is at the heart of medical practice and

is essential for maintaining trust and integrity in the patient-physician relationship. Knowing that their privacy will be respected gives patients the freedom to share sensitive personal information with their physician.

(World Medical Association, 2002)

The sharing of medical information is, of course, a central concern of ethics boards involved in overseeing biomedical research including biobanks. These bodies tend to have a range of rules to prevent access to medical information, requiring, for example, that researchers request informed consent again if they want to reuse the data for another purpose. However, these rules involve a range of caveats and ambiguities that mean that the issue of further access is open to negotiation on a case-by-case basis. If research involves 'minimal risk to subjects' and no adverse effect on rights or welfare of subjects (see Merz, 1997), US Institutional Review Boards can exempt it from the requirement for additional informed consent for future use. British Local Research Ethics Committees (LRECs) and Multi-centre Research Ethics Committees (MRECs) face similar dilemmas where biobanks are concerned. Following the 1998 Data Protection Act, the General Medical Council's (GMC) guidance on confidentiality was updated (2000), and it was argued that doctors should seek consent for every use, whether data was made anonymous or not, but this was heavily criticized by doctors because of its effect on disease surveillance and monitoring (e.g. cancer registries). The GMC now suggests that patients are told that their sample might be used anonymously for public health-related research and be given the choice to 'opt out' if they do not wish this to occur. The Medical Research Council's Operational and Ethical Guidelines on Human Tissue and Biological Samples for Use in Research (2001) also advocate anonymity and informed consent. The MRC guidelines state that, 'all personal information must be coded or anonymised as far as possible and as early as possible in the data processing,' but they also state that, 'generally, established collections can be used for research when samples have been made anonymous and there is no potential harm to the donors of the material, individually or as a group' (Medical Research Council, 2001). Given that the risks of biobanks are difficult to define, there is no consensus that this type of exemption procedure is acceptable here.

Genetic databanks raise other ethical dilemmas, given that the information they uncover might also be of relevance to family members and future generations. The Human Genome Organization (HUGO) argues that families should be allowed to access samples in exceptional circumstances:

Special considerations should be made for access by immediate relatives. Where there is a high risk of having or transmitting a serious disorder and prevention or treatment is available, immediate relatives should have access to stored DNA for the purpose of learning their own status. These exceptional circumstances should be made generally known at both the institutional level and in the research relationship.

(HUGO, 1998)

The Nuffield Council on Bioethics and the GMC have also taken this position. The HGC have unpacked some of the issues with reference to their principles of 'genetic solidarity':

> If the disclosure of information would enable the person to whom it is disclosed to take action to avoid a serious risk to his or her life or health, then it is certainly possible to construct a strong moral case for a person who is in a position to authorize disclosure. This is unless, of course, disclosure would have consequences which matched in seriousness the consequences of non-disclosure. An example of a situation in which there would be a strong moral obligation to authorize disclosure would be a case where there is a diagnosis of a form of cancer with a strong familial element. In these cases it would be difficult to justify opposition to allowing relatives to know of the advisability of testing . . . Such disclosure should be on the proviso that (1) an attempt has been made to persuade the patient in question to consent to disclosure; (2) the benefit to those at risk is so considerable as to outweigh any distress which disclosure would cause the patient; and (3) the information is, as far as possible, anonymised and restricted to that which is strictly necessary for the communication of risk.
>
> (Human Genetics Commission, 2002: 64)

This attempt to balance the risks and benefits of disclosure to family members seeks to prioritize the rights and wishes of the individual, only over-riding them when the situation is judged by medical professionals to be serious enough to warrant this. The notion of 'genetic solidarity' mediates individual interests and priorities, but these principles are to be negotiated through clinical practice: placing considerable responsibilities for the moral management of genetic information on health professionals.

These groups are, however, ambivalent about the best ways in which to manage the data in their charge, even if they are happy to rise to the challenges it poses. Concerns have been raised by some health professionals about the extent to which patients should be able to control their information, particularly when the public interest may be served by over-riding their right to confidentiality, for example, where health surveillance or criminality is concerned. Most legislation, including the UK Health and Social Care Act (2001), has a series of procedures in place to over-ride confidentiality in such cases, but these procedures have been criticized from a variety of angles. Some have suggested that they are too difficult to implement (see Verity and Nicoll, 2002), while others have argued the opposite (see Staley, 2001).

Other debates centre on the issue of access to data by commercial companies. Researchers and organizers with links to bioindustry tend to argue that biobanks should not be subject to strict confidentiality rules so that the information needs to be utilized by a broad range of parties in both the public and private sector to derive benefit. Its special significance for the health of future generations is also highlighted (e.g. Berg, 2001). Critics of such synergies have pointed to gene patenting controversies, such as that concerning Myriad Genetics' patent on the *BRCA1* and *2* genes involved in hereditary forms of breast cancer, as a reason why commercial access should be restricted (Rimmer, 2003).

Debates about biobanks also involve more technical disputes about the meanings of confidentiality and anonymity of the data. In order to assuage concerns about employers or insurers accessing sensitive information, and to conform to data protection laws, biobank data can be encrypted or made anonymous. Truly anonymous data loses some of its value to research of this nature, so biobanks tend to involve some sort of 'anonymised-linked format' (Barbour, 2003), using encrypted or encoded data. For example, Reilly and Page have criticized the US National Human Genome Research Institute's repository of DNA samples from 450 anonymous, ethnically diverse US residents, which was set up to conduct research into single nucleotide polymorphisms (SNPs), on the grounds that the irreversible severing of connections between individuals in the database and their ethnicity, sex and geographical origins, 'stripped this large repository collection of much of its scientific usefulness' (Reilly and Page, 1998: 15). However, security analysts have raised concerns about unauthorized access to the 'keys' that can unravel the codes and connections. They point out that biobanks tend to rely upon new data being added over time, thus compromising security. For example, Anderson has argued:

> The likelihood that unauthorized use will be made of information is a function of its value and the number of people who have access to it; and consolidating valuable private information such as medical records into large databases increases both of these risk factors simultaneously.
> (Anderson, 1999, referenced in Churches, 2003)

Confidentiality and anonymity are contested terms in both the public and biomedical arenas. This requires careful negotiation by the organizers and governors of biobanks, but the interpretive flexibility around these terms is less of a hindrance than one might imagine. Ambivalence creates a space for the actors involved with biobanks to negotiate their roles in mediating the 'public interest' dimension of biobanks and the construction of the rules and procedures of institutional ethics. Researchers and organizers have competing demands placed upon them, which requires negotiation about how to protect donors, and therefore encourage them to donate, and how to meet the demand for information from outside agencies with links to their funders and regulators. Doctors and scientists also need to defend their place in the public sphere, beyond the laboratory and the clinic, as respectable and trustworthy professionals who are not only capable of self-governance, but of acting in the best interests of the community, even when this might undermine their special relationship with patients and research subjects. This has resulted in a range of interpretations within the research community about where the balance should be struck between privacy and public interest, and a range of alliances with other interested parties such as government officials, patients' organizations and public interest groups. Genetic data gained from biobanking exist within a wider schema of preventative medicine, where agencies share information in the interests of the individual or, indirectly, the new public health. In this context, confidentiality or anonymity become something of a chimera, yet the focus upon them takes attention away from the political economy of surveillance of which biobanking is a part.

Leaving these concerns about other parties having access to genetic data aside, personalized feedback is actually quite popular with prospective donors to biobank research, and anticipation of this assumed benefit may be part of the reason that they have participated in the first place (Cragg Ross Dawson, 2000; People Science and Policy Ltd, 2002). Donors may also wish personalized feedback because of their sense of their 'right to know' information that is held about them, particularly when it might enable them to take steps to improve their health. These views were also expressed by members of the UK public who participated in focus groups where UK Biobank was discussed.[1] Others have also argued that information should be provided in the interests of health promotion. For example, patient groups who are keen to develop better surveillance of genetic disorders such as haemachromatosis, a genetic condition which is under-diagnosed, might argue that this information should be provided to participants, with appropriate counselling, so that they could take remedial action. This view is reflected in the European Convention on Human Rights and Biomedicine when it is argues that 'If it can prevent harm a person should be informed of unexpected findings of genetic analysis, if the information is of importance to treatment or prevention and even if the person has not asked for this information' (2001). Others have argued that this might breach a person's 'right not to know', a position reflected in the Human Rights Act, 1998 (see Staley, 2001).

Perhaps surprisingly, given the importance of individual self-management to contemporary health cultures, biobank participants do not tend to be given personal feedback about their test results, other than preliminary feedback resulting from the initial examination (such as blood pressure levels). The large scale of many of the new medical genetic databanks, the preference for encryption or encoding of subject's details and the focus on genes involved in common multifactorial conditions, means that such information is difficult to obtain. Other reasons which some researchers give against personal feedback include the lower standards of accuracy required of tests used in research rather than clinical circumstances, the ambiguity of research results and the lack of adequate genetic counselling. Researchers therefore tend to suggest alternative ways in which information can be fed back to participants, such as a regular newsletter explaining the progress of the research. This constructs participants as largely a passive, but supportive 'club' for the biobank, at once signalling and recognizing their shared altruism.

In this section, I have explored the flexible principles and practices which can be found when the confidentiality of data stored in biobanks is concerned. Tensions between the rights of the individual and the common good are negotiated in different ways by different parties involved with biobanks. Participants are variously treated as patients in need of protection and guidance, self-carers who actively contribute and respond to genetic research and disinterested research subjects. A diverse set of notions and practices around privacy and confidentiality create a space for professionals and other interested parties to negotiate the role of donors and researchers in clinical practice and institutional ethics – negotiations that are a form of governance in their own right.

Commercialization and governance

Although companies in the commercial sector also have their own genetic databases, their involvement in large-scale public projects is often said to be crucial to their success, given the high costs involved. As Wieting argues, 'communal goods are increasingly defined in terms of private interests', most notably in the rhetoric around the Icelandic Health Sector Database, where, 'deCode proponents see their project as embodying faithful adherence to the Icelandic historical tradition of enlarging the common good' (Wieting, 2002: 278). These arguments are also apparent in the research community in the United Kingdom, where, for example, Fears and Poste have argued that public–private partnerships are necessary to utilize the resources of the NHS (Fears and Poste, 1999) and that the deCode's exclusive licence is being used by some academics to 'stereotype and demonize' commercial companies, as 'insensitive to human rights' (ibid.: 268). The organizers of UK Biobank present the involvement of commercial companies as intrinsic to its success. As John Newton, the newly appointed CEO, argued at a recent UK Biobank Industry Consultation Meeting, organized by The Wellcome Trust, commercial application is in the public interest (4 April 2003).

Other critical commentators have raised concerns about how ethical review deals with potential conflicts of interests, particularly the interests of academics with stakes in commercial organizations. This is a special case of a more general concern about the conflicting values of universities, well characterized by Merz and colleagues as becoming 'schizophrenic', because they defend open and free sharing of ideas on the one hand, and pursue intellectual property rights and profit on the other (Merz et al., 2002: 968). This raises questions about the extent to which research agendas are shaped by the 'public interest' or the quest for profit, and the sidelining of so-called Cinderella diseases that affect small groups of people, so revenue from new treatments would therefore be low. However, questions such as these involve consideration of the priorities in health care funding and infrastructure, large and complex issues that cannot be addressed by L/MRECS, who act as important gatekeepers for research of this nature. Their duties when deciding about the ethics of research are to patients, rather than the public sector. This is an example of another way in which discussions of the political economy of biobanks are sidelined in professional domains in favour of the discourse of individual choice and progress in the fight against disease: two common tropes of late modernity.

Given the widespread coverage in the media of disputes about the patenting practices of pharmaceutical firms, and the prohibitively high costs of their tests and treatments for disadvantage groups, particularly in developing countries, commercial access to public resources have been brought into question

Box 6.2 Nationhood

Appeals to nationhood are particularly prominent in the discussions of the Icelandic Health Sector Database (see Wieting, 2002), but can also be found as a justification for commercial involvement in biobanking throughout the world. In the Lac-Saint-Jean region of Québec, the 'founder population', the 'Québécois de souche', is being studied by Galileo Genomics Inc, a Montreal company with links to US-based Myriad Genetics. Galileo's CEO, John Hooper, justified Galileo's agreements with a US firm in terms of its benefits to the Canadian economy when he said, '... if Galileo's founding scientists had not accepted the deal with Myriad they might well have ended up working there – most turned down lucrative US job offers before starting their own [Canadian] firm in May, 1999' (Staples, 2000: 118). Other countries' databases, such as the one planned by Singapore, are to be organized on the basis that they will make their data freely available to all academic institutions in their country, signalling a form of scientific nationalism (Cyranoski, 2000).

Others have raised concerns about commercial interests in genetic research undermining particular kinds of national or native identities. Concerns about DNA and nationhood are perhaps most pronounced in the case of first nation peoples, as evident in controversy surrounding the US-based Human Genome Diversity Project. Genetic researchers have collected the DNA from indigenous peoples around the world, and have been accused of 'biopiracy' for filing patent applications without any plans to share profits with the people on which the research is based. It is reported on the website http://www.ienearth.org/biodiversity.html that:

The US Secretary of Commerce filed a patent claim on the cell line of 26-year Guaymi woman from Panama in 1993. A wave of international protest and action by the Guaymi General Congress lead to the withdrawal of the patent claim in late 1993. The Department of Commerce also filed patent claims on the human cell lines of an indigenous person from the Solomon Islands. The patent claim was also later abandoned. The US Patent and Trademarks Office (PTO) approved patents on the cells lines of a Hagahai man from Papua New Guinea. The patents were granted to the US Department of Health and Human Services and the National Institutes of Health (NIH) in March, 1994. Once again, the patent holders faced public outcry and in late 1996, the NIH abandoned the patent.

(accessed 12 May 2003)

See also Indigenous Peoples Coalition on Biocolonialism www.ipcb.org

This type of research has also been criticized for reasserting racist notions of identity by undermining more diverse and fluid notions of nationhood that are based upon social and cultural communities, in favour of biological identities which are seen as fixed and somehow more 'real'. This raises particular concerns about discrimination against groups identified as having a higher propensity to certain diseases, because of their genetic heritage, reasserting old notions about the biological inferiority of certain races.

by a range of professional, patient and campaign groups concerned with genetics. Some have argued that industry has a moral obligation to share their profits and arrange preferential terms and conditions to the public sector and patient groups who provided the information that was required to develop their products. This has led some patient organizations to organize their own databanks, and to negotiate joint authorship and ownership of products arising from research that utilizes their material – for example, PXE International (see Merz *et al.*, 2002, for further details). As Merz and colleagues argue,

> [t]he patient community may not want a financial return, instead preferring to have an influence on access, pricing, and the terms guiding ownership and control of Downstream developments.

(ibid.: 969)

Pharmaceutical companies increasingly emphasize their ethical practice, and commitments to the public sector and the developing world. The obligations of the pharmaceutical and biotechnology industries are even recognized by one of its pariahs. DeCode have promised to pay expenses incurred by the Icelandic government in the setting up of their database. They will also pay the Icelandic government an annual fee, and 6 per cent of its annual pretax profits below a fixed amount, which would result in a net gain well above the annual health care expenditure if the company becomes profitable (ibid.). This is part of a growing trend of 'ethical capitalism', where companies protect their investments through cultivating good relationships with the media and the public at large, through activities such as the sponsorship of charitable trusts, including patients groups and taking part in public debates about the social implications of new technologies.

Donors' obligations are also extending beyond those of patients, to the obligations of citizens to participate in biobank research for the good of society. This brings other obligations to monitor and oversee the work of the professionals that are involved. However, the extent to which research participants would want to be so actively involved in research governance is far from clear; nor are the types of skills that they would need in order to be involved. Professionals have mixed views on who ought to be involved and on what basis. There are examples of professional alliances with patients' organizations with a specific interest in finding out more about their condition, for example in the case of PXE International and the Alpha-1 Foundation in the United States. However, when gene banks expand to include people with a diverse range of health problems the range of organizations that could be involved could grow considerably. Some professionals have argued that it is difficult to know how all of these groups could be involved on an equitable basis. As Merz and colleagues point out, there are many diseases for which limited or no collective representation exists, and even for those organizations that do exist, it is questionable to what extent they could be said to represent the views of everyone with the condition.

Others involved in these discussions are more positive about community involvement in biobanks, citing examples of medical research that have involved community representatives that could be relevant for gene banks. Sharp and Foster discuss one such study (2002) which involved representatives of the Akwesasne people collaborating with scientists from the State University of New York who were conducting research into the effects of certain chemicals found in the river on the health of people living along the St Lawrence River. This case is interesting because community members were involved in determining the goals of the project, and were involved in the project as research assistants, communicating results and sharing authorship on publications and reports from the research. Sharp and Foster suggest that this type of early and ongoing involvement of community representatives might go some way to mitigating the problems with anticipating the risks of this type of research. They note,

> ...it is precisely in those circumstances where collective risks are difficult to identify prospectively that the involvement of local study populations is most critical for minimizing potential harm.
>
> (Sharp and Foster, 2002: 147)

Researchers and organizers of biobanks must carefully negotiate the issue of public involvement in the current climate of distrust about their practices. Although full-blown public involvement such as that suggested by Sharp and Foster is unlikely to be viewed by many professionals as workable, there are other ways in which public engagement can be mobilized to encourage donations to biobanks and further use of the materials therein. Some have argued, for example, that public engagement through media coverage engenders a sense of shared priorities between research participants and medical researchers. This is well illustrated by the case of the MONICA project in Sweden, a study that investigated cardiovascular disorders and diabetes. Researchers approached donors 11 years after their initial donation to request consent for genetic research on their samples, and reported that only a very small proportion of participants did not give consent. Stegmayr and Asplund (2002) argued that 'people's readiness to contribute to genetic research is high, at least in the framework of a carefully conducted study that is well known to the population' (p. 635). Similar arguments are also associated with the ALSPAC study, which is known for its close involvement with donors.

These developments open up more space for inter- and intra-professional negotiation about the governance of new developments such as biobanks, constructing patients and publics as more active than before, but within a framework where professionals carefully control their involvement. Ethics is not, of course, purely a matter of public involvement or external oversight. At the same time as governance structures are blossoming, professionals' ethical discourse is also developing apace in other arenas. Genetics researchers articulate a strong sense of professional responsibility for the social and ethical implications of their work in number of professional and public domains. Researchers proclaim their professional responsibilities in publications where they stress the 'pre-analytical and post-analytical phases' of research (McQueen, 1998: 545), expressing their sense of duty to their patients, particularly patient confidentiality. As McQueen also argues, 'scientists and physicians have a collective moral and intellectual obligation to carry out research' (ibid.: 548).

Professionals have also expressed their criticisms of deCode and the Icelandic government in terms of their ethical, medical and scientific responsibilities, particularly their responsibilities to patients to respect the trust and loyalty on which their participation in research is based, in a variety of media (McInnis, 1999). As Pálsson and Harðardóttir point out, these discourses can be understood as a response to the structural changes in Icelandic health care, which has meant that physicians and scientists in universities are 'being removed from the discursive centre of local biomedicine' (Pálsson and Harðardóttir, 2002: 281) and wider structural changes within the Icelandic economy, notably the reorganization of fisheries. They are also part of an international discourse, where certain groups have much to gain from focusing attention upon the Icelandic situation as opposed to that of their own countries. Other professionals display their ethics, when, for example, they criticize the gene patenting practices of competitors to the Human Genome Map and their lack of openness in sharing genetics data, expressing their commitment to knowledge as progress, and a strong ethos of public service.

Governance is not simply a matter of structural control, but a means through which professionals and other actors negotiate their responsibilities concerning their work and its wider social relevancy. These actors invoke various discourses when constituting themselves as 'ethical beings', informally and formally, locally, nationally and internationally. These discourses concern the public and the public interest, social progress and perfect knowledge, as well as appeals to the sanctity of the individual (donor). At the same time as formalized structures of ethical review extend their reach into the institutions in which scientists work and the public arenas in which they also operate, and a wider range of experts are enrolled in the management these processes, professionals are engaging in ethics work in a more informal sense, in their discussions in the workplace and beyond.

Conclusion

The traditional model of biomedical research involves fairly distinct boundaries between donors and researchers, and commerce and the public sector: boundaries that imply different sets of rights and responsibilities for each of these groups. Donors are like patients: individualized and given rights. Professionals have the responsibility to protect these rights and to generate knowledge and ultimately social progress through their work, in alliance with the commercial sector. Risks are still largely defined by professionals and not open to negotiation, nor are the project protocol or outcomes. The public are collectivized, and largely passive, treated as a pool of potential recruits for the study, within a model of representative rather than participatory democracy. This model is based upon a strong notion of professional expertise in contrast to the lack of relevant expertise of the public, and, to a lesser extent, donors (who need to be sufficiently informed to give their consent). Health information is transmitted from individuals to their doctors, who analyse the information and ultimately facilitate product development that these individuals can then consume.

This model is, however, subject to a range of challenges and modifications in contemporary biobanking. The boundaries between all of these groups are becoming blurred, so much so that their rights and responsibilities are far from distinct. Notions of risk, social progress and consent all have to be negotiated by 'ethical beings', particularly professionals, but also self-carers and active publics whose own expertise can be construed as equivalent to professional expertise in certain circumstances. The extension of donors' rights emphasizes their individualism, yet the emphasis upon community and representative organizations emphasizes the collective. Notions of benevolent medicine and knowledge as progress are increasingly contested, although close community–patient–professional relationships still tend to be favoured on the basis that this will minimize risk, uncertainty and mistrust, and hence maximize social goods. Bureaucratic structures of oversight and professional self-governance are proliferating as concerns about risk and uncertainty grow. This should not be taken to suggest that professionals are necessarily more constrained than they were in the past, just that constraints have different forms and potential effects. Boundaries between professionals, companies, patients, families and communities are in flux rather than dissolved in these new arrangements.

Further reading

Merz, J., Magnus, D., Cho, M. and Caplan, A. (2002) 'Protecting subjects' interests in genetics research', *American Journal of Human Genetics*, 70: 965–71.

Pálsson, G. and Harðardóttir, K. (2002) 'For whom the cell tolls: debates about Biomedicine', *Current Anthropology*, 43:2, 271–301.

Sharp, R. and Foster, M. (2002) 'Community involvement in the Ethical Review of Genetic Research: lessons from American Indian and Alaska Native Populations', *Environmental Health Perspectives*, 110: suppl. 2, 145–8.

Staley, K. (2001) *Giving Your Genes to Biobank UK: Questions to Ask*. Report for GeneWatch UK, Buxton: GeneWatch, UK.

Tutton, R. and Corrigan, O. (eds) (2004) *Genetic Databases: Socio-ethical Issues in the Collection and Use of DNA*, London: Routledge.

7 Publics

Summary

In this chapter, I will look at the role of the public in genetics and society. I explore research into public opinions about genetics, criticizing the narrow ways in which people and their knowledge and understandings are conceived in this kind of research. I also look at other research into the public understanding of genetics that focuses much more upon the social contexts in which people come across genetics and give their views about its social and ethical consequences. Drawing on some recent findings, I will argue that although this work is much more sophisticated than public opinion research, the public are still represented in fairly narrow terms. Social researchers tend to position members of the public who they interview as citizens, but their research subjects often reposition themselves as other kinds of experts, and disassociate themselves from what they present as an ignorant and amorphous public. The ill-educated and fearful public remains a powerful notion in the contemporary governance of genetics.

Introduction

> Publics are queer creatures. You cannot point to them, count them or look them in the eye. You also cannot easily avoid them. They have become an almost natural feature of the social landscape, like pavement. In the media-saturated forms of life that now dominate the world, how many activities are *not* in some way oriented to publics?
>
> (Warner, 2002: 7)

A book on genetics and society would not be complete without some discussion of the roles of the public in relation to knowledge about and treatment of genetic disease. As I have argued throughout this book, discussions about new technologies like reproductive genetic tests, or new collections of genetic information like biobanks, tend to individualize the public, positioning them as potential patients or donors rather than social groups. When it comes to public policy, their input is also highly circumscribed. The public understanding of genetics is the main interest of professionals, policy-makers and academics in this area. Here the public or lay people become a mass of individuals, lacking expert knowledge in science or medicine, easily led by sensationalist media coverage, and largely apathetic about involvement in politics or policy decision-making.

Although almost two decades of work in the sociology of science and technology have undercut the theoretical and methodological foundations of this so-called deficit model, it is alive and well in the science communications industry and the policy communities it serves. As I shall argue in this chapter, the public opinion of genetics is still important in many policy discussions about new genetic technologies. More sophisticated and nuanced approaches to the public understanding of genetics, which blur boundaries between understanding and ignorance, expertise and laity, and publics and professionals, have also flourished. However, I will argue that the methodological tools and insights of this work can be easily adapted to tacitly support the deficit model. Although the focus nowadays is upon dialogue rather than knowledge deficits, efforts to build public trust have remained key to the ways in which policy-makers engage with public concerns.

Even the most radical approach to the public understanding of science involves an underlying vision of a consensual society, based around active citizenship and, in the words of Alan Irwin and Mike Michael, 'the belief that an open self-confident and self-critical society is a prerequisite for the successful management of scientific and social change' (Irwin and Michael, 2003: 154). This requires both knowledge and commitment on the part of the citizenry, in the interests of social progress. Such a formula implies that people would want to act in this way, if only they could see that it would be in their best interests. Active citizenship cannot be organized by the state, as this would undermine its very foundations. Nevertheless, the many social divisions and inequalities in modern societies radically curtail its potential to grow organically. Even if such a growth were possible, not everyone would have access to power and influence. As Warner has argued,

> The unity of the public ... depends on arbitrary social closure ... to contain its potentially infinite extension; it depends upon institutionalized forms of power to realize the agency attributed to the public; and it depends on a hierarchy of faculties that allow some activities to count as public or general and others to be merely personal, private or particular. Some publics, for these reasons, are more likely than others to stand in for the public, to frame their address as the universal discussion of the people.
>
> (Warner, 2002: 117)

In this chapter, I will explore the various framings of the public in what might be called traditional approaches to the public understanding of genetics, particularly opinion polling, and what Wynne has called constructivist approaches, which try to unpack rather than simply perpetuate dichotomies between lay people and experts, and their knowledge and values. I will consider how these approaches replicate, create and undercut social divisions in the process, and how this shapes the governance of genetics. Drawing on recent research, I will explore the ways in which the various methodologies in this area construct positions for research subjects which reflect a particular notion of how societies ought to function, and inadvertently perpetuate the divide between experts and lay people that they are designed to dismantle. I will argue that participants can actively resist the position of authentic citizen that researchers hope they will assume. Instead, they adopt a position based around expertise, be it technical or experiential. Researchers, policy-makers, and participants in consultation exercises all imagine publics. This imagining serves an important purpose, reinforcing their own sense of expertise and authority, on the one hand, and the expert-led system of policy-making, on the other.

Public opinion

Public opinion of biomedicine is increasingly of interest to policy-makers, funders and commercial companies. This comes at a time of mounting public disquiet about science and medicine. Large companies, charities and governments are increasingly concerned to avoid a public backlash and to secure the lucrative profits that can be generated in this realm.

However, this new significance of public opinion does not necessarily mean that the public's views are having more of an impact on policy-making and the practice of biomedicine. Instead, public opinion about genetics is largely an artefact, constructed through surveys or focus group studies. The public opinion that these polls construct is characterized as a social fact. However, what comes to constitute public opinion is largely divorced from the realities of people's daily lives. Surveys are often designed to access the views of representative cross-sections of the so-called general public. Interest groups are seen as unduly biased and atypical minorities so they tend to be excluded from such research, or, if included, treated as special, unusual cases. Surveys thereby ignore or 'exoticize' the views of special interest groups, particularly when they are critical of the official stance on the issue at hand. Davison and colleagues have questioned this tendency on the basis that such interest groups are better informed and more involved in the regulatory processes than ' "the public" at large' (Davison *et al.*, 1997: 332). They conclude

> Polling has become a tool not for engaging 'the public' in the business of public life, but for the creation of a simulacrum of politics.
>
> (Davison *et al.*, 1997: 330)

We must question any simple association between people's ability to be critical of biomedicine and how informed or knowledgeable they are, because this fails to capture what Irwin and Michael have rightly identified as the complex and rather diffuse ways in which knowing about technologies and supporting them are related (Irwin and Michael, 2003). However, Davison and colleagues have a point. Public opinion is very much an artefact of the polling process. As Pierre Bourdieu has noted, pollsters are 'past masters in the art of giving their customers accommodating answers tricked out with all the magic of a methodology and terminology that sounds highly scientific' (Bourdieu, 1990: 170). This results in statements reminiscent of cat food adverts, such as, 'three quarters of people interviewed are "amazed" by the achievements of science' and 'eight out of ten people agree that Britain needs to develop science and technology in order to enhance its international competitiveness' (Office of Science and Technology and The Wellcome Trust, 2000: 5). There is no discussion of when and why are people amazed by science, what science amazes them, or what it means to be 'amazed'. The general public are broken down and categorized to understand their views better: risk friendly and risk adverse, for example, or in the case of the recent Wellcome Trust survey, 'confident believers, technophiles, supporters, the concerned, not sure and not for me' (see Box 7.1).

Box 7.1 Attitudinal groups from the Office of Science and Technology and The Wellcome Trust (2000)

Confident Believers
Positive, self-confident and outward looking, the Confident Believers (17 per cent of the sample) tend to be interested in science because of the benefits it brings, and their interest in politics means that they tend to have faith in the regulatory system and believe that they can influence Government. They tend to be well off, well educated, middle-aged, and more likely to live in the south of Britain.

Technophiles
One-fifth of the total, this, the largest group, is confident, pro-science and well educated in science, but sceptical of politicians. They tend to be confident that they know how to get information when they need to, although they need reassuring that the regulatory system exists and works effectively.

Supporters
Some 17 per cent of the total, this relatively young group tends to be 'amazed' by science, engineering and technology and feels self-confident enough to cope with rapid change. They also tend to believe that the Government has got things under control. Although they, like everyone else, express most interest in the medical sciences, they tend to be slightly more interested in the physical sciences – especially engineering – than others.

Concerned

The Concerned is the smallest (13 per cent of the total) and most female (60 per cent) of the clusters. The Concerned have a realistic and positive attitude to life but are sceptical of those in authority. Their social grade, household income and education levels tend to mirror the population as a whole, but they tend to be rather home centred. They are interested in a whole range of topical issues, and they know that science is an important part of life, especially for their children.

Not Sure

This group (17 per cent of the total) tends to have the lowest household incomes, the lowest level of education, and falls into social grades D and E (semi- and unskilled manual workers, and those wholly dependent on state benefits). Their views tend to be unformed: they are neither 'anti-science' nor 'pro-science'. This is largely because the benefits of science are not always apparent in their daily lives, which are constrained by low income and educational achievement.

Not for Me

This group, 15 per cent of the total, mainly comprises those aged 65 and over, of social grade E women, and of slightly younger men of social grade C2 (skilled manual workers). Like the Not Sure group, they are neither particularly interested in political and topical issues nor in science. However, their lack of interest in science does not stop them appreciating its benefits for the future and its importance to young people.

Source: Office of Science and Technology and The Wellcome Trust (2000) *Science and the public: a review of science communication and public attitudes to science in Britain*, 6–8.

Although this is an improvement on the broad notion of a general public, these kinds of groups are far from sophisticated categories. They do not reflect the rich diversity of people's views and experiences; instead, they manufacture boundaries between particular 'groups', which are treated as if they were static. The public become a mass of individuals expressing their views. Individuals' 'personal attitudes' are fixed. Science and technology become a monolith, and distinctions between different forms of science, and different regulatory and commercial contexts are ignored. As Brian Wynne has argued, public opinion is thus objectified: stripped of its relational qualities. Groups like these inevitably caricature, despite their stated aim to the contrary. They miss the diversity, ambiguity and dynamic qualities of people's views, and, crucially, objectify opinion, decontextualizing it from people's day-to-day lives.

Of course, relationality and context are not the concern of people in the science communications and polling industries. Their interests lie in mobilizing public opinion facts in public discussions and debates about the future of science and technology policy. These groupings only make sense when we consider the reason for their construction. In this case, it is explicitly stated that the purpose of the groupings is to determine how best to effectively engage different groups in scientific issues – or in the words of the Wellcome report, so that 'Hooks can be identified...to...attract people to take a more active interest in science and scientific issues' (Office of Science and Technology and The Wellcome Trust, 2000: 66). An 'amazed public' would undoubtedly boost the Wellcome Trust's ongoing campaign to get the government to spend more money on science and technology and to counter public disquiet about new developments such as cloning and xenotransplantation. 'Don't knows' are of less use, and therefore interest, as Bourdieu puts it,

> [d]on't knows are the trauma, cross and misery of polling institutes which endeavour by all means at their disposal to reduce them, minimize them, even to conceal them.

> (ibid.: 172)

One way of ensuring more answers is to construct respondents as citizen-consumers. As biotechnology moves closer to the market, questions about it are framed in terms of health behaviour and activity rather than public policy. For example, 'Would you allow your child to have gene therapy in order to treat a genetic disease?' is asked, rather than 'Should money be spent on gene therapy research as opposed to improved care for people with genetic diseases?' The dangers of gene therapy experimentation (especially given the recent high profile cases of suppressed evidence of deaths during gene therapy trials), or the commercial environment in which technologies such as these are being developed, are not open for consideration.

The public's acquisition of facts and information tends to be measured in opinion polls about science and technology. Indeed, what is often being studied is the public misunderstanding of science not the public understanding of science. This is what is called the deficit model of science. Although this has been roundly criticized by scholars such as Wynne and Irwin, and it is rejected by leading figures in the arena of public understanding of science, such as John Durant and even Lord Sainsbury, the British Minister for Science, its influence remains pervasive. Technical know-how is privileged over an appreciation of the social, cultural and political contexts in which science takes place, and people never have enough of it. Experiential knowledge tends to be treated as secondary to formal scientific knowledge. Knowledge is often cast as a set of facts and figures, which is objective and neutral, and can be given to people to increase their understanding.

Low levels of technical knowledge are often correlated with the public's emotions, gut-reactions, subjective knowledge, psychological constructs, and fears of science and technology, which are considered to be background

Box 7.2 MORI genetics poll shows public's confusion, 12 March 2000

An alarming 65 per cent of adults in Britain are confused and unclear as to what is meant by the term 'gene cloning' according to a recent MORI poll...

However, 74 per cent of the public agrees that gene therapy is acceptable if tightly controlled, once the process was explained to them...

Overall, attitudes to gene cloning and gene therapy are overwhelmingly more positive than negative despite the fact that many knew little about these processes before taking part in the survey...

Commenting on the survey, Action Research's Director of Communications and Marketing, John Grounds said 'More needs to be done to cut through the media's sensationalism and instead focus on the importance of genetic research and its role in the vital work that Action Research and other organizations fund'.

misconceptions. Such misunderstandings can be linked to low levels of knowledge. Another favourite strategy is to measure levels of public acceptance, and then to marvel at how high it actually is, despite low levels of knowledge. Media sensationalism is the cause of the public's confusion or lack of understanding about genetics. The conclusions drawn from surveys like these are often about how to improve public understanding and, by implication, acceptance of science. A good example is a MORI poll commissioned by Action Research, a medical charity (see Box 7.2).

As Brian Wynne has pointed out, little or no attention is paid to why the public know what they know, or about what they might like to know. The importance or relevance of particular information to their life is under-recognized, as are their perceptions of the usefulness of knowledge. The question of whether or not there is any point in people knowing a lot of technical information when they are unable to influence the direction of scientific and medical research or activities is not considered.

Davison and colleagues also note how measures of support can be manipulated by the survey design. Questions can be framed in a way that minimizes the risks associated with new technologies and emphasizes their benefits in order to demonstrate greater support. For example, Genetically Modified Organisms (GMOs) can be compared to older practices such as fermenting and selective breeding, to emphasize their similarities with safe and reasonable practices and therefore their acceptability. A classic example of the actual measurement of this effect is a survey carried out by MORI for Novartis, a biotechnology company, which measured the 'approval rating' for various scientific developments, including cloning and xenotransplantation. MORI explicitly recognizes that approval can be increased by particular question

Box 7.3 Increasing public support for controversial technologies

Q: Which, if any, of the following do you support and which do you oppose?

	Support (%)	Oppose (%)	D/k (%)
Scientific experiments on live animals	31	60	8
Cloning of animals such as Dolly the sheep	16	74	9
Cloning and growing human cells	28	60	11
Genetic modification of plants	20	62	16
Genetic modification of animals	16	71	11
Human genetic testing for diseases	66	20	11
Human to human transplants of organs	90	6	3
Animal to human transplants of organs	44	42	13

Q: Which of the following would you support or oppose if it was proved necessary to achieve a permanent cure/vaccine for Alzheimer's disease?

	Support (%)	Oppose (%)	D/k (%)
Scientific experiments on live animals	48	43	9
Cloning of animals such as Dolly the sheep	35	57	8
Cloning and growing human cells	46	43	10
Genetic modification of plants	42	47	11
Genetic modification of animals	37	54	9
Human genetic testing for diseases	75	17	8
Human to human transplants of organs	85	10	6
Animal to human transplants of organs	50	39	10

Source: MORI (1999).

frames. They even make a virtue out of such a finding (see Box 7.3). As press release from MORI states,

> Without an application being stated, the approval rating for scientific experiments on live animals was only 31 per cent. When asked the same question in connection with a permanent cure or vaccine for Alzheimer's, the approval rating increased 17 points to 48 per cent (with 43 per cent opposed)...
>
> 'Novartis is very encouraged by these results. We believe biotechnology will enable us to deliver health, environmental and commercial

benefits, for example new medicines and environmentally sustainable options for modern agriculture'.

(MORI, 1999)

Measures of public acceptance can clearly be manipulated by the way questions are framed. Although this is sometimes recognized by pollsters, it does not lead them to a developed, more reflexive and open survey designs, but is identified as a useful tactic for increasing public support for science.

In these types of surveys, it is the public who are being problematized, not science. The focus is often narrowly topical, about particular technologies to do with health or the environment. As Davison and colleagues note, little attention is paid to the political economy of science. The surveyors and their sponsors are not really interested in what people think about these issues, indeed, they would probably prefer that the public did not think about these matters at all. 'Science' is narrowly defined, as neutral and objective, with overwhelmingly positive applications. It is also presented as easy to control, with proper regulation. Scientists are represented as responsible professionals, with the public good as a principal motivator, not commercial profit. When commerce is discussed (usually in relation to food production), the emphasis is upon science providing consumers with more and better choices.

The risks and benefits of science are also presented in a particular way that emphasizes the neutrality of science and take attention away from its wider social and political context. As I have already argued, benefits are frequently highlighted and risks are often downplayed. However, the types of risks and benefits that get attention also frame the science and technology in a particular way. Science and technology are presented as products, chosen by rational consumers. A narrow form of utilitarianism underpins these frameworks. For example, respondents might be asked to weigh up the pros and cons of new genetic technologies in terms of their usefulness – identifying criminals and curing disease, versus breaches of confidentiality and discrimination. Respondents inevitably end up valuing the benefits, and agreeing that the potential disadvantages are minimized by effective regulation and ethical practices. Yet, this model of how risks emerge and are controlled is highly artificial, a point which the public intuitively recognize in other contexts where they are able to express ambivalence and concern about new technologies, experts and their governance (Kerr *et al.*, 1998b,c; Eliasoph, 1998).

Greater public support for new developments remains a key motivator of a lot of research into the public opinion about genetics. In a typical survey, the public are cast as citizen-consumers. Minority opinions are marginalized in favour of the majority. People's opinions are treated as if they were a product of their level of understanding of technical details. Little attention is paid to why people access particular forms of knowledge or what it means in the context of their daily lives. Results are easily manipulated, to produce positive conclusions, emphasizing the neutrality and objectivity of science, its benefits, and the optimal balancing of its costs and benefits. These exercises have little to do with democracy and empowerment of the public, and are closely associated with 'manufacturing consent', stifling dissent and promoting the interests of commerce and industry.

Lay knowledge

In contrast to the market research genre of public opinion polls, a significant body of work on lay knowledge has been built up over the last 15 or so years. Often based upon in-depth interviews or focus groups, this work often challenges the deficit model of public understanding of science.

Researchers adopting what Wynne calls the constructivist model of public understanding of science argue that many different groups make up the public, and that their knowledge is not simply a matter of technical detail, but involves a broader understanding of scientific practices and institutions. The constructivist model looks at how peoples' social locations shape their understanding of and engagement with science. Social location takes account of a range of characteristics like age, race, gender and class, as well as other things like people's health experiences and that of their families, the community of which they are a part, and their educational and work histories. All of these things shape how we come to understand science in general, and genetics in particular. People hold their own 'stock of knowledge', to use Schutz's term. This is a product of their experiences, which are both unique and culturally shared. Their interpretation and response to science is shaped by this stock of knowledge. This will variously affect how confident people are about engaging with and challenging scientific evidence and arguments, how seriously they view disabilities and their treatments, and their attitudes to genetic testing and to health professionals. The situations in which people are located also shape the ways in which they respond to new genetic technologies, both positively and negatively.

In research following the constructivist model of public understanding of science, the public are treated as socially located actors, rather than either a general mass, divided along basic lines of gender and class, or grouped according to simplistic caricatures like 'technophile' or 'not for me'. Special interest groups are taken seriously, not marginalized. Knowledge and understanding are seen as complex, socially embedded activities. For example, Parsons and Atkinson (1992) and Lambert and Rose (1996) have done studies of lay knowledge of genetic disease, based on in-depth interviews with people who have a genetic disease in their family, and have found that people reinterpret complex medical information in the context of their day to day lives. This determines what information they find relevant and how they make sense of that information. Parsons and Atkinson show, for example, that people translate statistical risk information about their chances of having a child with a genetic disorder into definitive yes or no answers in order to make sense of its meaning. Similarly, Lambert and Rose show how people operate with what they consider to be a 'good enough' level of knowledge about their health, which is shaped by a range of experiences with family members, professionals and media. Wynne and colleague's work on risk perception illustrates how, in the words of Turner and Wynne, 'risks are defined primarily according to their perceived threat to familiar social relationships and practices and not by numerical magnitudes of physical harm' (Turner and Wynne, 1992: 122). They emphasize the 'rationalities of everyday life', which means that risks are not narrowly defined, but relate to perceptions of the institutions and organizations involved with defining and controlling those risks, so trustworthiness of professionals plays an important role in how people perceive technologies old and new. As Wynne notes,

> Understanding may mean the ability to use technical knowledge effectively, but inability to use such knowledge does not necessarily mean lack of understanding, Understanding science may also mean understanding its methods rather than its specific content...and it may mean understanding its institutional characteristics, its forms of patronage and control, and its social implications.
>
> (Wynne, 1995: 363)

In relation to genetics, people's technical understanding involved basic ideas about heredity and disease, and varies depending on their education and experiences. People do not have to have formal qualifications to have technical knowledge. For example, parents of children with genetic diseases like cystic fibrosis can be very knowledgeable about the disease, because they had to find out about it to help their child. However, people do not have to have a high level of technical understanding to be able to discuss issues around genetics and health in a sophisticated manner (see Kerr *et al.*, 1998b,c). People's discussions might involve the expression of concerns about the acceptability, or otherwise, of research and clinical practice that is actually taking place, or could take place in the future. A focus on the technical deficiencies in what they say obscures other important aspects of their accounts. The sophistication of the discussion is not necessarily compromised by inaccuracies in some of the technical details. Moreover, where people explicitly recognize their own absence of scientific knowledge this can also involve sophisticated discourses of ambivalence about their dependency upon and/or lack of trust in official knowledge-claims. Their appreciation of the irrelevancy of particular knowledge to their own lives, or the explicit alignment of expert knowledge with expert responsibility also becomes apparent (see Irwin and Michael, 2003). In the case of genetics, this might involve the expression of concern about the fallibility of genetic testing, and its iatrogenic effects (risks created by the tests themselves, like miscarriage in the case of amniocentesis), and the difficulties of scientific proof. Their discussions might address institutional practices, for example competition and cooperation among scientists, sources of funding, especially the role of pharmaceutical companies and government, and the relationships between geneticists and the media.

These types of knowledge form the terrain of public engagement with genetics, which is more about the application of science in the face of uncertainty, and the body language of scientific institutions and scientific professionals, than it is about the precise details of particular technologies. More formal scientific knowledge does not simply mediate against these types of concerns, quite the opposite sometimes occurs (Evans and Durant, 1995).

In direct contrast to opinion polling, the constructivist model of the public understanding of science problematizes science rather than the public. The aim of this type of research is not to improve or increase the public understanding of science, but to take the public's views seriously and to consider how best to incorporate them into policy-making. Science is not treated as if it were neutral or objective, scientific evidence is not a series of unproblematic facts, and the way in which science is organized and performed is crucial to discussions about how effective and appropriate it actually is. People engaged in constructivist studies have found that the public understand this well enough, but traditional methods of accessing their opinion fail to give them the opportunity to demonstrate and develop this understanding, as it is not considered to be relevant.

Another important feature of the constructivist model of public understanding science that is worth mentioning here is its methodology. In-depth interviews or focus groups tend to be used in this approach, in contrast to quantitative surveys. There is nothing intrinsically constructivist or interpretive about qualitative methods. However, when used within an interpretive framework, in-depth interviews and focus groups have the advantage of allowing participants to express their views in an open environment. Interviewees can, to a certain extent, set agendas and raise issues that they think are important. The researcher's analysis can also be fed back to participants for comment, which can then be used to enhance the study results. This approach treats participants as active research subjects, not objects to be dispassionately analysed. Their views are seen as a product of the interview process, not as some pre-existing, fixed set of responses which an interview will tap, so analysis of the transcripts takes into account the context in which the accounts were expressed, and how this has shaped them. Finally, this kind of approach highlights ambiguity and contradictions in people's accounts, rather than manufacturing consensus. Altogether, it generates a much richer and more challenging data set than surveys and other studies adopting the deficit model.

Active citizenship

The constructivist approach to the public understanding of science is also linked to a series of more recent consultation and public involvement exercises based around notions of active citizenship, especially in Europe. A variety of public scandals, about mad cow disease, organ retention and genetically modified organisms, have intensified governmental efforts to engage more fully with public concerns about new science and technologies. As Beck argues, 'hazards exacerbate the dependence of everyday life on science, but they simultaneously open the scientific monopoly on truth to public discussion' (Beck, 1995: 161). Prestigious scientific institutions such as the UK's Royal Society, began to adapt in the face of what was perceived to be widespread public mistrust of science. This involved greater commitment to transparency and openness, and a range of consultation exercises influenced by the qualitative approaches of constructivist public understanding of science. As Irwin and Michael (2003) stated, such exercises were quite explicitly tied to an agenda of building public trust, as the following quote from the House of Lords Select Committee on Science and Technology report entitled, 'Science and Society' indicates

> Policy makers will find it hard to win public support on any issue with a science component, unless the public's attitudes and values are recognized, respected and weighted along with the scientific and other factors.
> (House of Lords Select Committee on Science and Technology, 2000: 6)

The Department of Trade and Industry's White Paper, entitled 'Excellence and Opportunity: A Science and Innovation Policy for the 21st Century', continued this theme, focusing upon 'confident consumers' and the importance of 'public debate'.

There are, however, a number of problems about how publics' and citizens' identities are constructed and framed in these types of exercises (Dunkerley and Glasner, 1998; Irwin, 2001). Irwin (2001) has argued that in one such exercise – the British Government-led initiative, Public Consultation on Developments in Biosciences (PCDB), conducted in the late 1990s – consultees were positioned as *re*active rather than as active citizens, engaging with the science on terms which were set by the institutional partners behind this initiative. Irwin's claim is supported by the House of Lords Science and Technology Committee who took the view that the PCDB was more market research than a genuine public consultation, and was more 'professionally led' rather than 'citizen-led' (Irwin, 2001: 13). This is despite the organizers' original promise that the consultation was supposed to give people influence over the future of science.

As Petersen and Bunton (2001) and others such as Dunkerly and Glasner (1998) have also commented, this framing of members of the publics' entitlements to participation in genetic policy-making can slip into a sense of their obligations to participate. The public are supposed to engage in informed debate in order to stem the potential for abuse of genetic information. Yet there remain very few routes for members of the public to influence the types of research and legislation that are developed.

It is also often the case that not a wide cross section of people who are being consulted in these exercises, but special interest groups, such as patient organizations (Rabeharisoa and Callon, 2002). Avowedly rejecting the paternalism of an earlier period, these groups work within an 'ethos of consumer involvement' (Petersen and Bunton, 2002: 193), actively seeking influence over research agenda and public policy through partnerships with the commercial sector (Rabinow, 1999; Fleischer, 2001). These groups are well positioned within the governance processes of Western democracies. A good example is the Human Genetics Commission Consultative Panel – made up of people affected by genetic disorders. Many of these people act as lay representatives at public meeting organized by the Commission and other similar committees, alongside business people and representatives from public-interest groups. Typically, meetings like these are not widely publicized in advance and participation tends to be by invite only.

A range of qualitative techniques such as focus groups has been used to promote active citizen involvement in this area. However, focus groups also position publics in particular ways. They create a space for people to engage in moral reflection and to articulate or indeed construct a range of fears and concerns, often in response to hypothetical, futuristic scenarios. It is not, therefore, surprising that the participants' accounts are dominated by the use of common tropes from popular culture, as they discuss these issues. Professionals are, in contrast, often positioned in different ways, more often than not as individuals rather than members of groups, as specialist interviewees who are informing and guiding the interviewer because of expert knowledge. There is less space for professionals to explore a range of past and future scenarios when they are interviewed in this way. Even when given the opportunity to engage in more open-ended dialogue, professionals might choose not to pursue these lines of argument, taking a more individualistic and instrumental approach to their involvement in research or consultation, again often based on their role as experts and educators. These different types of interviews open up space for different types of reflection, which, when compared, can give the impression that the public have more concerns than professionals, and are more likely to be influenced by the discourses of popular culture than professionals. This can reinforce rather than undermine the lay–expert divide.

Citizens' juries and consensus conferences are another way of engaging the public in science. These have long been favoured by public interest groups critical of patenting, nuclear power and other big sciences such as GMOs. Towards the end of the 1990s, they were adopted by a range of more traditional agencies such as the Consumer Council, the Royal Society and The Wellcome Trust, as they moved away from the so-called 'deficit model' of public understanding of science towards public engagement, transparency and dialogue.

The Institute of Public Policy Research (IPPR) developed its model for citizens' juries in the United Kingdom following the design of similar models in the United States and Germany (Stewart *et al.*, 1995). The IPPR worked with several health authorities, piloted five citizens' juries on matters of health care policy. As Lenaghan notes,

> Since 1996 citizens' juries have become an established method for public involvement, with over 30 taking place in the UK, endorsed by government and the subject of continuing interest and innovation.
>
> (Lenaghan, 1999: 50)

A citizens' jury consists of between 12 and 16 jurors who are recruited by sampling, to be broadly representative of their community. They are brought together with moderators to address an important policy issue. Jurors are then briefed about the background to the question, through written information and oral evidence from witnesses. They can cross examine the witnesses and organize various small discussion groups to aid their deliberation. The jurors' conclusions are written up in a report that is distributed to relevant parties. Usually the people who commissioned the jury have undertaken to respond to the conclusions within a set time, but their recommendations are not binding.

One example of a citizens' jury is the area of genetics is the Welsh Citizens' Jury, organized by the Welsh Institute for Health and Social Care, commissioned by a large transnational pharmaceutical firm who had not made a commitment to act on the jurors' recommendations. The jury were asked to consider the question, 'What conditions should be fulfilled before genetic testing for people susceptible to common diseases becomes available on the National Health Service (NHS)?' None of the witnesses was from an ethnic minority, or groups opposed to genetic testing, and questions have been raised about the representativeness of the jurors with respect to disability (Glasner, 2001). The jury endorsed the use of genetic testing for single gene disorders, and made a number of recommendations. For example, they suggested that the National Health Service should take the leading role in the provision of genetic testing services, and that a family history should be taken from every new patient registering with a primary health care team in order to identify those at high risk. They also argued that the general public and politicians need to have a better understanding of the implications of genetic testing (Welsh Institute for Health and Social Care, 1998).

Citizens' juries such as this one can also exacerbate the lay–expert divide, perhaps unwittingly. There is considerable evidence that jurors are capable of digesting and applying scientific knowledge and bringing rich and sophisticated appreciation of their own and others' personal experiences to their deliberations, as well as learning from their experience as a juror (Einsiedel, 2002). This is often seen as justification for the use of this method: a reason to celebrate rather than denigrate lay expertise. However, this focus upon the opinions of the jurors takes attention away from the ways in which expert witnesses participate in the citizens' jury process. Their position within the exercise remains relatively fixed and unreflexive. They largely function as repositories of knowledge and advice. Theirs is an exalted role, no matter how much attention is given to the sophistication of the juror's decision. Experts' subject-positions can therefore be black boxed by the very process of subjecting expert knowledge to public scrutiny. Citizens' juries are also particularly susceptible to the guidance of experts involved in steering groups, and in the moderation of their deliberations (Glasner, 2001). Lack of familiarity with the protocol and the subject matter, combined with close contact with moderators with whom jurors build relationships of trust, also shapes the ways in which they come to articulate their concerns. As Glasner notes,

> Key actors may establish juries as part of a sophisticated public relations exercise. User involvement becomes a technology of legitimation. It can also become a token in the armoury of more powerful champions... translated as 'playing the user card'. This suggests that an important role for juries may be educational and consultative rather than the promotion of active citizenship.
>
> (Glasner, 2001: 44)

Constructing citizens and publics

This chapter began with a critique of opinion polling, exploring the ways in which this type of research uncritically perpetuates certain models of science as neutral and the public as ignorant. However, we must also question the models of science, citizens and publics underlying notions of lay knowledge, constructivist public understanding of science and active citizenship. The extent to which people come to participate in focus groups, consensus conferences, constructivist technology assessment, and the like, as ordinary members of the public is open to question.

Close analysis of dialogue at a range of public–professional meetings and conferences and in more intensive focus group discussions with groups of people from a range of backgrounds, suggests that people often position themselves as different from the so-called general or ordinary public, by mobilizing other relevant expertise in their accounts.[1] For example, some participants in a focus group with members of a local Friends Meeting House did not tend to position themselves as citizens but as people with expertise in a range of scientific, legal, and business fields, as did members of public interest groups and patient or support groups, despite the fact that greater public involvement in decision-making was one of their stated objectives. In contrast, these participants often positioned the public as amorphous, ignorant and largely powerless. It seemed that member of the public was not a position that many people wished to occupy. Voter or consumer or patient were, however, more acceptable positions, even for people who were principally positioned as scientific or medical experts, so long as they were given the space to shift between these positions. Participants seemed to be more open to exploring these different roles when they were friends, colleagues or members of particular groups. However, as Eliasoph has forcefully demonstrated, people's circles of concern shrink when they speak in any public context and this can mean that in group contexts 'informal etiquette made some political intuitions speakable, and others beyond the pale of reasonable, polite discussion' (Eliasoph, 1998: 7). In wider public fora, such discussion is even less easy or acceptable, given that people's positions as expert speakers or as members of the audience are often fixed through the event's format and agenda which means that they would have to be disruptive to adopt alternative positions.

These difficulties with taking up a citizen's role in these types of discussions are exacerbated by the predetermined agendas of many consultation exercises, which do not speak to the genuine concerns of many ordinary people, who simply do not get to decide what sorts of questions are worth discussing. The fetish for consultation about genetics, as opposed to less glamorous topics such as affordable housing or respite care, is but one example of this seques-tration of experience (Smith, 2002). Some people are nevertheless more able to move between subject positions more easily than others are, mixing expertise and personal experience, even in highly public events. Disability activists are, for example, able to display scientific and medical understandings, and to appeal to morality and political actions based upon notions of justice and rights, but they are also able to tell personal tales of their own experiences of disability and impairment. This form of identity politics uses discussion about the body, emotions and relationships to challenge the denial of public exis-tence that so many disabled people experience. For people for whom such flex-ibility is afforded, positioning as an ordinary member of the public would, however, be improbable. Indeed, one might go so far as to say it is precisely because of a lack of ordinariness about these speaker's experiences that their movement between subject positions becomes possible.

We must also consider the case of the professional lay person in order to fully understand the dynamics of public involvement with genetics. This type of person tends not to be found in highly public spaces such as open meetings or conferences. Instead, they attend meetings where audiences and speakers are invited. They also take on positions in a range of sites of con-temporary governance, particularly ethical review panels that must now have a token lay person in order to function. Lay here often translates into a rela-tive of patient. For example, the ALSPAC Ethics and Law Committee has two lay members described as lay members and ALSPAC mothers. Other lay members might be trustees of charities, as is the case with the Steering Committee for the UK Stem Cell Bank and for the Use of Stem Cell Lines, one of whose lay member is an ex-trustee for the Parkinson's Disease Society, or journalists, as is the case with the second lay member of this committee, who is also a manager for a Health Care Trust. Once appointed, lay members can take on a professional role, in the sense that they become experts at being lay members. They learn the appropriate etiquette for how to draw on a par-ticular set of knowledge and experience that is considered lay in relation to the topic at hand, but expert in another context. Nursing, journalism, busi-ness and charitable work constitute acceptable domains from which to con-struct this lay status. Given that the remit and domains of these committees intersect, lay members can be recruited to other committees, enhancing their status as professional lay members.

These various roles for lay people in contemporary genetic governance are highly circumscribed, and often inhabited by people who claim a right to participate on the basis of their expertise and relationships in the social networks which influence policy-making in this area (including media, business and charities). When subject positions are more flexible, people often avoid taking up the role of ordinary member of the public. This means that opening up a space for public dialogue often involves a corresponding reinforcement of experts' status as they are called upon to inform the public, or answer their questions, rather than engage in sustained reflection about their own role or status in relation to the topic at hand. Exercises in public involvement or engagement with genetics tend to be organized by influential public and professional bodies, and follow formats and agendas with little space for boundaries between expertise and laity, or knowledge and values, to be breached. Highly circumscribed by the political and economic circumstances in which they are conceived, these exercises hardly constitute democratic decision-making.

Unfortunately, scholars in the social studies of science and technology seem to have lost sight of these various means by which publics are constructed in the dialogic models that they have fostered, and, indeed, in the theories that underpin them. In much of the more recent sociology of science concerning expertise, the publics are constructed as idealized citizens or lay experts (I write here as a perpetrator of this very notion – see Kerr *et al.*, 1998c).

Harry Collins and Robert Evans (2002) have recently published a wide-ranging critique of this kind of work. They argue that the focus upon extending the domain of decision-making to a range of publics, has created a 'problem of extension', that means 'there are no longer any grounds for limiting the indefinite extension of technical decision-making rights' (Collins and Evans, 2002: 235). The current preoccupation with the lay expert brings with it a certain naïve relativism about experience and knowledge according to Collins and Evans, making it difficult to decide what types of knowledge and experience are more valuable in solving problems of public significance. Collins and Evans question the common contention that public participation redresses elite domination of technical decision-making, and begin to explore what aspects of people's relationships with the topic at hand qualify them to contribute to decision-making in a meaningful way. This leads them to set out a normative theory of expertise, including technical expertise, interactional expertise (a specific level of technical expertise within a specific technical specialism) and contributory expertise (enough expertise to contribute to the science of the field being analysed). They distinguish this from lay expertise or the public as a whole, whose contribution they view as less valuable.

Although their solution to the problems they identify can also be criticized for its relatively conservative reassertion of the lay–expert divide, they do raise an important point when they query the extent to which lay expertise has been reified and idealized by scholars in the field. Collins and Evans are, I think, right to deconstruct the notion of the lay expert, and to criticize its role in social studies of science. As this work becomes increasingly divorced from empirical study, analysts tend to romanticize about the lay public. For example, Shiela Jasanoff's response to Collin and Evan's original article, involves the following bold statement:

> ...expertise is constituted within institutions, and powerful institutions can perpetuate unjust and unfounded ways of looking at the world unless they are continually put before the gaze of laypersons who will declare when the emperor has no clothes...participation is an instrument for holding expertise to cultural standards for establishing reliable public knowledge, standards that constitute a culture's distinctive civic epistemology...participation can serve to disseminate closely held expertise more broadly, producing enhanced civic capacity and deeper more reflective responses to modernity.
>
> (Jasanoff, 2003: 398)

One cannot disagree with the democratic impulse behind this statement, but the extent to which laypersons can ever function in this way is, as I have argued earlier, severely limited by the roles and functions ascribed to them, even in consultation and engagement exercises which try to empower them. When given the chance to inhabit roles of their own creation, people often choose to take up an expert rather than a lay position, which begs the question: to what extent is the lay persons' gaze an idealized construction of the analyst rather than a genuine part of these types of scenarios? I would suggest that it is not lay persons who declare that the emperor has no clothes, but other experts, be they patients, lawyers, journalists, science/health activists or even sociologists.

A similar idealism can be found in Wynne's work, when he argues that 'proper participants are, in principle, every democratic citizen and not specific sub-populations qualified by dint of specialist experience-based knowledge' (Wynne, 2003: 411). Wynne constructs these idealized citizens despite his stated concern to expose the 'presumptive imposition of such meanings (and identities) on those publics and the public domain' in other's work (Wynne, 2003: 402). However, as I have argued, democratic citizen is a subject position that many people do not want, or are unable, to inhabit. Even those who adopt this mantle, veer between a range of identities that cut across or sometimes undermine the position of democratic or ordinary citizen.

I do not mean to suggest that Collin and Evan's typology is free of these problems of idealism, as they too fail to account for how people move between and beyond the categories of expertise that they have mapped. Their solution to 'the problem of extension' of decision-making is also far too conservative. They offer a different set of reasons to support citizens' juries and constructivist technology assessment, rather than a critique of the problems therein, especially what we might call 'the problem of expert co-option' of these types of exercises, sometimes to pre-existing expert-led agendas, at other times through the subject positioning of the participants themselves.

Conclusion

In this chapter, I have reviewed the main ways in which the public tends to be positioned in relation to genetics, by researchers and policy-makers alike. I have argued that a lot of emphasis continues to be placed on the public's lack of understanding, or trust in genetics. Qualitative research with a more sympathetic approach to people's views of genetics shows that people often have sophisticated understanding of genetics, even when not directly affected by genetic disease. This has contributed to the reshaping of the so-called deficit model of public understanding of science to a newer dialogue model. The public is now consulted about policy matters in a more sensitive and respectful fashion. However, many flaws and inequities remain. These newer methods of consultation can all too easily be turned to the agendas of the more powerful commercial and governmental bodies who commission them. The ways in which experts and publics are positioned in exercises designed to give the public a greater say can subtly reinforce rather than undermine the divisions between them.

Categories of publics and experts are no longer taken for granted by many scholars and researchers involved with the public understanding of genetics. Consultation exercises that promote understanding and trust between a broad range of stakeholders in genetic science are a vast improvement on the old-style deficit model of public opinion polling. However, these newer approaches can subtly reinforce the divisions they claim to be dismantling, not least, because participants are so accustomed to valuing expertise, however contested and frustrating that might be. Researchers too have a stake in perpetuating their own expertise and authority, and forging links with the policy community is an important means by which this can be achieved. This is not to say that everyone involved in accessing and interpreting the public understanding of genetics are simply motivated by base self-interest. However, it would be naïve to assume that the dynamics of social status only involve the participants, rather than the organizers and commissioners of these exercises. The ways in which these groups construct the public can never be divorced from these processes.

Further reading

Irwin, A. (2001) 'Constructing the scientific citizen: science and democracy in the biosciences', *Public Understanding of Science*, 10: 1–18.

Collins, H. and Evans, R. (2002) 'The third wave of science studies: studies of expertise and experience', *Social Studies of Science*, 32: 235–96.

Warner, M. (2002) *Publics and Counterpublics*, New York: Zone Books.

Wynne, B. (2003) 'Seasick on the Third Wave? Subverting the hegemony of propositionalism: response to Collins & Evans (2002)', *Social Studies of Science*, 33:3, 401–17.

8　Futures

Summary

In this chapter, I analyse various discourses of the future of genetic medicine
and the ways in which these discourses reinforce certain contemporary practices and values, while challenging others. I examine these twin discourses of
future cure and future risks in discussions about a range of potential genetic
technologies – gene therapy, genetic enhancement and cloning. I consider
how ideas about liberty, enlightenment and perfection, and their twins, coercion, risk and dissolution, are manifest in variety of documents about future
genetic technologies. I look at the ways in which these imagined futures are
framed in relation to present and past practices, and consider what shapes the
production of these discourses. I am especially interested in the overall effect
of these twin discourses of cure and risk upon our collective sense of ownership and control over these new technologies. Discourses do not simply
reflect prevailing cultural norms and values: they shape them too. However,
there are many different sets of values and norms within contemporary society, reflected in the considerable ambivalence about the future of genetics and
science more broadly. This means that the effects of future discourses are
always partial and contingent upon a range of social processes.

Introduction

The new genetics is replete with images and discourses of a perfect future,
where genetic diseases are preventable and genetic enhancement can optimize
an individual's potential for success. Advocates of these new developments
draw sharp distinctions between the past and the future, and how their critics
erase them. These invented futures can be found in a variety of popular science accounts, but they also exist within the more sober accounts of bioethicists, scientists and government. A futuristic thread also runs through much
of the contemporary discussions of gene therapy, just as it did in the past
when eugenicists fantasized about breeding supermen. Discussions about
gene chips, tailored medicine and genetic profiling also involve a strong discourse of future potential. Alongside these optimistic scenarios, there are

more dystopian visions of the future, where a genetic underclass emerges, or genetic surveillance becomes commonplace and infringements of privacy and personal freedom proliferate. The dangers of cloning, including deformed babies, premature ageing and fractured identities, are also raised. These negative versions of the future are often thought to be the product of sensationalist journalism. However, they can also be found in social and ethical discussions in which health and science professionals play a key role.

Recent work on the sociology of the body has emphasized the importance of the utopian telos of perfect bodies in contemporary society (Chrysanthou, 2002). Transparent, informed bodies are marketed by the health promotion industry. This encourages contemporary citizens to turn their gaze inwards, to improve themselves. Many have embraced this culture of self-promotion and surveillance, experiencing it as a form of freedom, rather than oppression as: 'biological identity becomes bound up with more general norms of enterprising, self-actualising responsible personhood' (Rose, 2001: 18). However, there is much confusion and controversy about the benefits of this quest for perfection, with many arguing that it breeds neuroticism and fatalism, stoking uncertainty while promising certainty (ibid.). As Caygill notes, there is a sense in which the dialectic of enlightenment means that promises of liberation inevitably create new forms of subjection (Caygill, 2003). This is a powerful theme in the critiques of authors such as Dorothy Nelkin, who have suggested that limitless consumer appetite for gene enhancement technologies will lead to a genetic underclass, whose genetic endowments will be forever inferior (Nelkin, 2001).

These paradoxes and ambivalences has resulted in a series of compromises between the aspirations of professionals and fears of publics, and discourses of the future are one means by which this is negotiated (Caygill, 2003). As Brown *et al.* have noted,

> Like all discourses, 'the future' is constituted through an unstable field of language, practice and materiality in which various disciplines, capacities and actors compete for the right to represent near and far term developments.
>
> (Brown *et al.*, 2000: 3)

As Levitas (1990) has argued profound conflicts of interest generated by the new forms of ownership in contemporary biopolitics, shape these discourses of the future. However, this does not necessarily involve radically different notions of technology and social progress. As Richard Ashcroft has noted, advocates and critics of 'post-human futures,' such as designer babies and genetic enhancement, share a discourse of market liberalism which seriously limits our exploration of new genetic technologies and their political and policy contexts (Ashcroft, 2003).

I begin my analysis by considering a recent government document on the future of genetics in the United Kingdom. Although the futures presented therein are less striking than those of the more speculative genres of futuristic thinking, they give important insights into how new genetic technologies and their potential impacts are being constructed, and shaped by policy-makers and funding bodies. I go on to explore a range of future-discourses produced by bioethicists from across the political spectrum, considering the context in which they were written and the ways in which they could influence policy agendas, and clinical practice. I then compare these various visions of the future with the ones that some health professionals have produced, and with those of the popular media. I explore the similarities and differences in their approaches and ways in which their visions close down and/or open up discussion and debate about the technologies of the present and how they might be developed.

Policy-speak

The British Government's recent white paper, 'Our inheritance, our future. Realizing the potential of genetics in the NHS' (Department of Health, 2003), frames genetics in terms of a series of revolutionary discoveries, which will be applied to prevent disease through 'personalized medicine' provided by the NHS. The paper proposes a series of investments in basic research and the development of infrastructure in order to provide these future services. The main premise is this:

> A greater understanding of the part played by our genes in the development of disease will result in a step-change in disease prevention, diagnosis and treatment. The Government's vision is for the NHS to lead the world in harnessing the potential of genetics in healthcare and for NHS patients to benefit from the safe, effective and ethical application of the new genetic knowledge and technologies...
>
> We are looking to the future. Over time, we will learn more about the genetic features of common diseases such as heart disease and diabetes... There will be the option to test people for a predisposition to disease, or a higher than normal risk. Treatment, lifestyle advice and monitoring aimed at disease prevention could then be tailored appropriately to suit each individual...
>
> Advances in genetics will lead to new drugs and novel therapies.... Gene therapy holds out the prospect of new treatments for a wide range of common conditions...
>
> The exact timing for different genetic advances is uncertain and it is too early to accurately predict all our requirements for the next decade. But unless we act now to ensure we have firm foundations to build on, the NHS will be left trailing...
>
> (Department of Health, 2003: 4–5)

The white paper places a lot of emphasis upon the benefits of these technologies, not just to individuals seeking to control their own health futures, but also to the British economy and even the NHS, which will benefit from the inward-investment around these technological developments. The white paper suggests that, in order to accommodate these developments, the skills and expertise of professionals need to be increased so that they can explain these new choices to patients. The Human Genetics Commission is represented as a group of independent experts who will play an important role in this process, providing advice and easing public anxiety about the implications of these developments. Human reproductive cloning is firmly rejected, but so-called therapeutic cloning, which involves research on embryos grown in culture and their destruction after 14 days, is not discussed.

The white paper sets up a variety of distinctions between past and present, public and private, expert and citizen, and technology and society. These distinctions can be found in many of the scientific and medical discourses on future cures. As I have argued throughout this book, there is little acknowledgement of the expertise of patients and citizens, or critical engagement with the choices of professionals in much of the literature on genetics and society, and the white paper is no different in that regard. It prescribes very limited roles for patients, the public and the majority of front-line health care professionals in the genetic services of the future. Their responsibilities are to accommodate and understand these new technologies, not to participate in any kind of decision-making about whether or not they should be developed in the first place. In the white paper, advances in scientific knowledge alter society, but society does not influence scientific knowledge. This remains pure and neutral: nature uncovered.

We can look to other analyses of the policy process to help us to understand how such a document comes to be produced. As Cambrosio and colleagues (1990) note, a range of bureaucratic norms and standards will have shaped its production, none of which are specific to science and technology, or even genetics:

> Defined by a set of intra-governmental tasks and constraints, a central problem being that of disposing of representations of the external world in terms of internal representations of governmental action.... Government action plans are not limited to a representation of the world as it presently is; they also aim at prospecting and, more importantly, constraining the future.
>
> (Cambrosio *et al.*, 1990: 200–14)

The white paper was produced, in part, to demonstrate that the British government has a vision of future genetic services. It was important to demonstrate their commitment to capitalize upon and stimulate future British investment in genomic research, in order to reassure the science community. It was also important to reassure health professionals about the future of these services within the NHS, at a time of growing disquiet within their ranks about commercial genetic testing and the implications of gene patenting for testing within the NHS.

A significant amount of background negotiation would have taken place during the production of the paper, specifically with representatives of the NHS and genetics research community. This would have been necessary to translate the concerns of these so-called stakeholders into the final document. The discourse of cure is enrolled in this process, forming an important interface between the political, scientific and medical worlds through which the document was constructed.

The white paper's advisory committee are likely to have played a part in these processes. From a total panel of fourteen, six members are very senior physicians, with positions of authority in a range of professional bodies and genetics institutes, and considerable experience as members of other regulatory bodies. Three are industry representatives, two represent patient groups, one of which has considerable links with industry and actively campaigns in favour of genetic research and screening. One genetic counsellor is represented in the group. Baroness Onora O'Neill, an important figure in the committees and commissions where the ethics of biomedicine are discussed, and Professor Sir David King, the Chief Scientific Adviser are the other members. The members of this committee do not have clearly defined interests that we can simply trace onto the final document, nor do they simply represent well-defined groups with obvious interests in common. They nevertheless had a privileged access to discourse production in the way that other groups, such as the disability community, have not. This is reflected in the emphasis upon cure and progress in the final document.

Other groups who are likely to have shaped the paper include important scientific institutions such as the Royal Society. Indeed, the Royal Society held a series of public meetings called 'People's Science Summit' around the time the paper was being written. Sir Paul Nurse raised the possibility of genetic identity cards for babies at one of these meetings. Although both speaker and participants were highly sceptical about such developments, the white paper notes that the government has asked the Human Genetics Commission and the National Screening Committee to consider the case for storing the genetic profiles of newborn babies. It has been rumoured that a leaked paper from the BioIndustry Association also shaped this proposal. Informal relationships between government, industry and the scientific establishment have clearly also shaped the questions which are raised in the white paper as well as the solutions it proposes. However, this commitment to investigating the social implications of developments such as newborn genetic profiling before, rather than after, the technologies are developed, seems rather hollow, given that this is not a serious proposition for many science and health professionals. In highlighting this issue the white paper sign posts the government's commitment to ethical oversight through bodies such as the Human Genetics Commission, but retains an emphasis upon technological development in other supposedly less controversial areas, such as gene therapy, biobanking and reproductive screening.

The document would also have been important in legitimating the status of the various groups charged with its development and implementation, including the genetics division of the Department of Health. It would also have played a part in building and reflecting important networks between government departments and other agencies, emphasizing their shared priorities and policies. The white paper refers to other authoritative sources such as the Human Genetics Commission and the Nuffield Council on Bioethics on several occasions to demonstrate these ties with relevant stakeholders. It signals the governments' expertise and control of the future of genetics, and marks out key alliances with professionals in the scientific and medical sectors, while also signalling a responsiveness to potential unease about these arrangements in the form of an acknowledgement of public anxiety.

Imagine that the white paper had recognized the social context in which these technologies are designed and used, and taken fuller account of the ambivalence and tensions around, for example, intellectual property rights, the value of this research into cures and treatments, or people's uptake of any resultant tests. This would have made it a much more provisional document, and opened a space for dialogue and criticism from other interested parties which would, at the very least, stall some of the investments announced therein. This could be seen as a failure of political nerve, and it might encourage resentment and concerns among the medical and scientific professions at a time when there is already considerable disquiet about structural changes to the NHS and lack of funds for scientific research. The cure motif, and the attendant reductionism of many of the white papers' proposals, avoid many of these problems, while also presenting a broad brush agenda for future research and service provision that only loosely ties the government into these developments.

Of course, we must be wary of exaggerating the extent to which government policy documents such as this white paper drive genetics research and service provision. This paper discusses investments in the range of £80 million, a small amount, relative to the investments of pharmaceutical and biotechnology companies in this sector. However, these proposals will shape the direction of at least some genetic research, and they contribute to a positive ethos around the science that indirectly shapes practice in this area.

Public bioethics

A very different genre of future discourse also exists in what Kelly usefully calls public bioethics (2003). Public bioethics involves a range of public debates and discussions about biofutures. These occur alongside the deliberations of the committees and commissions of institutional bioethics who are charged with exploring and regulating the ethical implications of new technological developments. Public bioethics tends to be dominated by a small number of high profile bioethicists, particularly in the United States. Their debates and discussions take various forms, notably articles in specialist magazines, popular science books and talks at public debates.

Leon Kass, whose article 'Ageless bodies, happy souls: biotechnology and the pursuit of perfection' (2003) I will review shortly, is typical of the conservative element in these discussions. Kass considers the philosophical implications of the future of genetics, and takes a cautious approach to the risks they might bring. An influential figure in US bioethics, he is currently the Chair of the President's Council on Bioethics, a body that President Bush has charged with evaluating stem cell research and cloning with respect to the sanctity of life. He is a well-known conservative, who has long raised objections to abortion, cloning and euthanasia.

Kass's article begins by evoking the golden age of biotechnology, while going on to acknowledge that ongoing anxieties are also valid, given current instabilities, such as terrorism, and past efforts at social control. Kass highlights concerns about man playing God or post-human futures as the most important of these worries, given their implications for the meaning of humanity. Although he acknowledges that concerns about enhancement may be remote from public policy agendas, he stresses the importance of considering these trends, given that 'the push towards bio-engineered perfection' is 'the wave of the future, one that will sneak up on us before we know it, and, if we are not careful, sweep us up and tow us under' (ibid.: 2).

Kass goes on to consider some of these potential futures, noting that the technologies that they might involve have not been explicitly created for the purpose of perfecting post-human beings but for the purposes of prevention and cure. However, he states that the profound human urge to improve, and the commercial environment in which these technologies are developing, mean that these 'techniques and powers can produce desires where none existed before, and things often go where no one ever intended' (ibid.: 3). Focusing upon 'self-improvement', particularly 'ageless bodies' and 'happy souls', Kass notes the fuzzy boundaries between notions such as therapy and enhancement and argues that the distinction between them is not helpful when trying to establish an ethical framework for acceptable practice. He outlines a variety of objections to these technologies: concerns about safety and risk, unfair advantage to enhanced individuals, and social control. However, he downplays many of these concerns on the basis that life is full of risks and people ought to be able to choose between them, but that inequalities of access are inevitable. The central question for Kass is about the goodness or badness of the thing being offered. He suggests that three human goods are of central concern: 'the goodness of the ends, the fitness of the means and the meaning of the overarching attitude of seeking to master, control and even transform one's own given nature' (ibid.: 7).

Kass locates concerns about 'men playing God' as an effort to retain a sense of life and the world as a gift, and to position subjects as modest, restrained and humble in the face of this world. He argues that concerns about the means by which perfection might be achieved are about protecting the 'normal character if human beings-at-work-in-the-world ... which when fine and full constitutes human flourishing' (ibid.: 11). Kass is concerned that transformations remain intelligible, so that we have a sense of ownership over them. He accepts procreation, human renewal and an element of psychic pain, and rejects the pursuit of perfect bodies. In Kass's view, we ought to know our place within the generations and accept mortality. We should revel in authentic pleasures, evade anxiety and attain true happiness.

Although obviously very different from the white paper, Kass's article involves a similarly naïve view of technology and nature. Technology, for Kass, seems to drive certain social relations because it fulfils the human instinct and desires for perfection. Kass encourages his readers to resist subjugation to these drivers, in favour of another form of subjugation to the holistic, natural world and, implicitly, God. His dystopian vision is of a future scared by inappropriate enhancements, which will ultimately reduce rather than add to the sum of human happiness.

Kass side-steps difficult social and political analysis in favour of metaphysics. In true conservative fashion, democratic decision-making, regulation, and restrictions on markets are rejected, while the power of God is applauded. Biomedical technologies are seen both as demonstrations of human instincts, best kept unchecked, and a way of creating even more problematic desires. The public are largely passive in the face of these new developments. These views are reflected in many aspects of institutional bioethics, particularly in the United States where conservative values are in ascendance. They are also reflected in the corridors of academe, where the public are imagined as especially lacking in technical and philosophical insights. These values will undoubtedly have shaped the vision of the future that Kass presents here. However, his account also has a role in fostering certain impressions of genetics and society rather than simply reflecting them. Kass is engaged in bringing God back into the increasingly secular enterprise of bioethics. He is also involved in raising the profile of the committee that he chairs, and in documenting his views so that they are recognized as legitimate parts of policy considerations in this area.

Glen McGee's approach to *The Perfect Baby* (1997) is more liberal in its tone and prognosis. He represents a more radical element in public bioethical discussions about biofutures, although it is certainly not a minority position. McGee is part of an influential group of bioethicists at the Center for Bioethics, University of Pennsylvania. *The Perfect Baby* is a best-seller. McGee has acted as an advisor to numerous state commissions, federal committees and private companies. He is a leading advocate of stem cell research and gene patenting. He is close to the director of the Centre, Arthur Caplan, who is listed on his website as one of the top fifty most influential people in American healthcare, and is clearly one of the key actors in the political and institutional governance of genetics in the USA.

McGee proposes what he terms a 'pragmatic' approach to the ethics of genetics, 'where practical wisdom is privileged' above what he calls

'GenEthics'. For McGee,

> the answers scientists need to develop research and clinical priorities and the answers parents need in order to make difficult decisions, are found in the contexts of good science and good parenting.
>
> (McGee, 1997: ix)

This leads McGee, like many in this field, to argue that 'the use of genetic means to improve humanity is dangerous, but no more morally problematic than the use of piano lessons, mega vitamins and expensive private school' (ibid.).

McGee works towards this position via his own form of discourse analysis of the 'hype' and 'fears' around genetics, which he argues are largely based upon misinformation. He argues that this rhetoric has little saliency in the world of the clinic, castigating critics, such as Jeremy Rifkin for idealizing nature and demonizing technology, and criticizing advocates, such as Leroy Hood, for unconstrained genetic determinism. McGee diagnoses a problematic rift in popular consciousness, where outlandish fears and naïve genetic determinism are stoked by lack of scientific understanding. McGee goes on to argue:

> Only by replacing determinist, reductionist thinking with a pragmatic recognition of the interaction of the biological and cultural matrices can we begin to develop coherent accounts of organic function, which both acknowledge the power of genetic structures and do not obscure their reciprocal, temporal relationships with the environment.... These relationships find their meaning in the lives of parents who must make the most important choices about uses of the new technologies...each of whom wants a healthy, happy, 'perfect' baby.
>
> (ibid.: 78)

This leads McGee to advocate a cautious approach to new genetics tests, until a clear account of their efficacy can be produced and understood by expectant parents. He argues that physicians should be seen as providers of services, and dismisses non-directive counselling as dishonest. McGee also advocates regulation to eliminate genetic discrimination, and is strongly in favour of scientific governance such as peer review. However, McGee makes a strong argument for genetic enhancement, on the grounds that the drive for self-improvement is worthy, and that genetic enhancement is likely to have a small overall effect upon the population, given that they are bound up with a much more mundane set of parental concerns. He advocates tolerance of other people's decisions, supportive parenting and diffuse hopes, rather than overbearing and hasty judgements.

Although McGee engages much more fully with the social and technical context of genetic interventions than many of the writers in this genre, he also strongly associates genetic technology, or more particularly knowledge, with progress, and unquestioningly promotes advanced liberal capitalism when he stresses the ethos of service provision, client choice, and self-improvement. He also maintains the boundary between experts and lay people in his discourses of public ignorance and fear, and perpetuates rather than unpacks rhetorical appeals to good science or everyone's desire for a perfect baby. Despite his convincing deconstruction of critiques such as that of Jeremy Rifkin, McGee does not engage with a more diverse and sophisticated array of criticisms of genetic technologies that do not depend upon idealizing nature or demonizing science, and do raise penetrating questions about how scientists and society decide what constitutes good science, or, indeed perfect babies. Instead, he is content to leave the first set of questions to the scientific community, and the second to parents. Despite his claim to the contrary, McGee does not really engage with the ways in which these decisions come to be made, although this is part of some of his later work in other areas.

McGee's thesis is a critique of the more abstract work of authors like Kass, as discussed earlier. He rejects metaphysics in favour of pragmatics. He argues that professionals and their clients ought to be able to make decisions, free of regulatory interference. He wants to keep both God and Nature out of these decisions. He reflects the secular, professional approach to governance, but nevertheless seeks to carve a place for bioethics in these processes. His arguments are designed to reinforce prospective parents and health care professionals' sense that they have a right to autonomy and control over their individual futures.

This takes attention away from the range of financial, professional, institutional and parental pressures which shape the kinds of services that particular clinics provide, and influence how their standards of services are constructed, that is, how good screening is defined and evaluated. Parents may be encouraged to use new screening or therapeutic technologies in order to raise the profile of particular clinics, or justify and give credence to controversial research. This may be presented in the media as 'their choice', but it is far from being truly informed and freely made. The questions that many professionals and parents are grappling with concern the ethics of these types of relationships and their implications for future children. However, these questions do not tend to be part of the discourses around biofutures, even McGee's.

Richard Ashcroft has identified similar trends in his deconstruction of the Fukuyama–Stock debate about the biomedical futures of human beings. Fukuyama and Stock are key players in US public bioethics and, as Ashcroft notes, they often perform in public debates across Europe and the United States to promote their respective books: *Our Posthuman Futures* (2002) and *Redesigning Humans* (2002). These debates attract considerable media attention, framed as they are around the potential for radical transformation and major risks to humanity. Fukuyama's position parallels Kass's when he emphasizes the dangers to human dignity, wrought by new genetic technologies such as genetic engineering. He nevertheless takes a wider perspective on political economy when he notes the dangers of instability and violence resulting from uneven distribution of genetic benefits and burdens, particularly between developing countries and the rich West. He favours regulatory controls to prevent the development or application of technologies which he sees as threatening human dignity, a position which Ashcroft notes is understandable, given his recent appointment to the US President's Council on Bioethics (alongside fellow conservative, Kass).

Stock is much more enthusiastic about genetic futures, presenting what Ashcroft neatly summarizes as 'a vision of unlimited human improvement in the free market, with decidedly sceptical views on the power of national or international regulation to control innovation' (Ashcroft, 2003: 59). This leads Ashcroft to diagnose a form of technological determinism in both positions, which is not based in the technology *per se*, but in human nature, with its unlimited and basic impulses to improve our own, and our off-springs' futures. He argues that both Fukuyama and Stock:

> subscribe to the mainstream view in US politics, which is that there are limits on the capacity of the state to improve human nature; limits which are set by human biological and psychological nature.... [sharing] a discourse of economic and quasi-economic interests as the drivers of technological, social and species change.
>
> (Ashcroft, 2003: 59)

It is particularly striking that they both focus on what is by now a standard list of future technologies and their potential benefits, including increased longevity, reduced suffering, enhanced intelligence and beauty, within an idiom of consumer choice. Their focus is upon the diseases and preoccupations of the rich. They give little consideration to biofutures where the sum of human happiness in increased through people's enhanced capacities for empathy or benevolence.

These types of futures are, of course, deliberate exaggerations, in order to make them more interesting to a general audience. They also reflect one of the discursive styles within the disciplines of theology and philosophy, where the extreme consequences of particular developments are deliberately constructed by the author as a means of exploring and evaluating the directions that are available in the present. Of course, such discourses do not directly shape the direction of research and regulation, but they are far from divorced from these processes. They contribute to the public imagination, perpetuating certain notions of individuality, agency and control, which, in turn, inform policy-making, albeit implicitly. The very fact that some of the key authors in this arena are members of advisory bodies that influence regulation suggests that a certain premium is being placed upon the wisdom of their views, at least in some circles, if not others. The predominant focus upon individual choices within the context of market liberalism, and the interpretation of technological trajectories as the outcomes of the human instincts of progress and perfection, narrows the expectations of policy-makers about the extent to which they can shape technological developments and regulate their consequences. This places responsibilities for morality and justice with consumers and patients, and responsibilities for safety and efficacy with the people who design, build and market these technologies, undermining a discourse of shared responsibilities for these values and practices.

Biomedicine

Public bioethics intersects, to some degree, with the discourses of future cures in biomedicine. Bioethicists write in both domains, but physicians and scientists also write about ethics when they consider the potential developments in their field. Researchers with a keen interest in the ethics of their work often attend public meetings where these futures are discussed, and engage with the work of authors like Stock and Fukuyama. These are some of the ways in which researchers in this controversial field act as 'ethical beings'. This is simply a matter of representing themselves to a perceived sceptical public (although this cannot be dismissed as irrelevant). It is also part of their professional identities. Engaging with ethics in these ways allows professionals to negotiate the complex demands and expectations bound up in their work. It allows them to retain a sense of the bigger picture in the face of highly specialized and narrowly focused work. Ethical reflection allows them to negotiate their role in relation to fellow workers and other parties with which they must interact in the course of their work – patients, regulators, funding bodies and journalists, to name a few. Scientists and health professionals express a range of positions on what constitutes ethical research and service provision, which leads some to criticize and others to accept various popular writers' versions of genetic futures.

Turning to consider the discussion of future cures and their risks in the bioscience and biomedical literature, a variety of common themes are apparent. Authors in these publications tend to focus their attentions on the safety and efficacy of these technologies, casting this as a matter of ethics. Much of the discussion centres on reproductive cloning, germline gene therapy and genetic enhancement, and it is a paper about the ethics of these developments that I will discuss here.

David Resnik, a philosopher and bioethicist, and Pamela Langer, a molecular biologist, have co-authored several papers on the ethics of human germline gene therapy, one of which appeared in 2001 in the journal *Human Gene Therapy*. In this paper, they argue that 'procedures that could be construed as "genetic enhancement" may not be as morally problematic as some have supposed, once one understands that the boundaries between therapy, prevention, and enhancement are not obvious in genetic medicine' (Resnik and Langer, 2001: 1449). This, they argue, means that human germline gene therapy may be the 'medically and morally most appropriate way of avoiding the birth of a child with a genetic disease in only a small range of cases' (ibid.) They discuss a range of ways in which boundaries between 'prevention' and 'enhancement' are blurred in the medical encounter, stressing uncertainties about the time of onset of genetic diseases. Eugenics is dismissed as intervention at the level of the gene pool, not the individual (i.e. human germline manipulation will not affect the gene pool if it is used in only a few cases). The authors normalize genetic interventions, by drawing comparisons with other 'socially acceptable medical interventions' that prevent or alleviate the effects of ageing. After rejecting general arguments against germline manipulation, the authors argue that each technology must be evaluated on a case-by-case basis, like McGee. They state,

> If we accept the idea that 'disease prevention' and 'life prolongation' are morally legitimate reasons to develop or implement a medical procedure, then we must ask, 'What methods are the best ways of achieving these goals?'
>
> (ibid.: 1453)

This involves understanding the risks and benefits of particular procedures. They ask a range of questions to help with this task, including 'Is the procedure more risky than pregnancy itself?' concluding that, 'One of the most convincing arguments for using what they call Human Germ Line Genetic Manipulation (HGLM) is that it may offer a small set of parents their only hope of procreating genetically related children who are free from severe genetic diseases' (ibid.: 1454).

Other articles about genetic enhancement in the biomedical and scientific press take a similar stance. For example, Jon Gordon (1999) stresses the importance of 'sensible guidelines for developing policies governing human genetic enhancements', based upon knowledge about 'exactly what we are doing' when we intervene in the human embryo (ibid.: 2023). This leads him to dismiss current efforts at gene transfer as 'scientifically unjustified' (but not morally unjustified). Placing his faith in the scientific and medical community, Gordon argues that attempts to ban gene transfer would be too cumbersome because it could infringe the privacy of patients, and the freedom of research. Informed consent and risk–benefit analysis are more effective breaks than legislation, although, 'irresponsible use of technology can never be stopped, even by legislation' (ibid.: 2024). Gordon ends by arguing,

> Gene transfer studies may never lead to successful genetic enhancement, but they are certain to provide new treatment and prevention strategies for a variety of devastating diseases. No less significant is the potential for this research to improve our understanding of the most complex and compelling phenomenon ever observed – the life process. We cannot be expected to deny ourselves this knowledge.
>
> (ibid.: 2024)

This emphasis upon knowledge as a form of enlightenment, intervention as a matter for individual cases, and ethics as a matter of risk–benefit analysis, is common throughout this genre. Although these authors come to a range of positions on the acceptability of particular research initiatives and procedures, which means that their outlook is far from hegemonic, their focus upon the individual and the particular tends to take attention away from the broader political, economic and social circumstances in which these technologies might come to proliferate. Bioethical discussions in biomedical and scientific journals often work notions of individual choice, consumer demand, technological progress and perfection, into rationalist, positivist scenarios of cost–benefit analysis, translating 'ethics' into safety and efficacy, in the same way that many of the commentators and regulators of biobanks represent these projects. This places enormous faith in rationality without considering the extent to which notions of safety and efficacy are open to multiple interpretations in clinical contexts. The rhetorical link between knowledge and progress is also common throughout science and medicine, as are representations of diseases in terms of suffering, devastation and fear. People's desire for genetically related children and the removal of problem genes are simply assumed. For both critics and advocates alike, gene manipulation technologies tend to be presented as a response to parental demand, rather than a matter of professional development.

Mass media

A discussion of the discourses of genetic futures would not be complete without consideration of the ways in which new genetic technologies are represented in the mass media. The media is often criticized for exaggerating both the benefits and the potential risks of developments such as genetic enhancement, gene therapy and cloning. Cloning received considerable press coverage in the wake of the announcement of the successful cloning of Dolly the sheep in 1997. As Sarah Franklin has argued,

> Dolly became a kind of totemic animal, a sign of the times, a millennial sheep, not only because her birth was considered to be biologically impossible, but because her birth became a symbol of the transgressive potential of the new genetics more generally – a potential we could describe as anti-foundational in its capacity to disrupt taken-for-granted limits formerly assumed to be incontrovertible and all but self-evident.
>
> (Franklin, 2001: 336)

This makes cloning an ideal topic for analysis of the use of metaphors and imagery in popular accounts of genetics. Nerlich and colleagues have studied the use of dystopian imagery in popular discussions of human cloning. They argue that 'the discourse on cloning is based on a network of metaphors and commonplaces' (Nerlich *et al.*, 1999: 1.15), which generate fears and hopes about cloning among the public in such a way that 'the fictional representations of our biological future have merged with scientific facts and photos: fiction has become flesh' (ibid.: 2.4). Frequent mentions of Dr Frankenstein, and Brave New World pepper these accounts. In their sample, the discourse of reason was mobilized by the scientific community, notably scientists at the Roslin Institute where the work took place, to counter what its proponents constructed as exaggerated fears of the future, including rich cloners, replacement children and armies of Elvises. In so doing, the scientific community reproduced, and to some extent perpetuated, the metaphors they set about debunking.

Other press coverage concentrated upon the reactions of some of the figure heads of public bioethics, as discussed earlier, notably Lee Silver whose book *Remaking Eden: Cloning and Beyond in a Brave New World* (1997) unashamedly constructs a biofuture with many ideas and devices from science fiction. This links to the so-called discourse of doom, which focused upon the abuse of cloning technologies by rich and powerful anti-heros, such as Saddam Hussein. Another public scientist with a taste for the extreme was also at the forefront of these accounts – Richard Seed, who planned to offer cloning to infertile couples, working with the Raelian cult.

Although they present a useful tour through some of the more colourful media discussions of cloning, Nerlich *et al.* do not spend much time considering the models of human agency, responsibility and governance that underlie these various discourses. They also appear to assume that these discourses are, largely, adopted and regurgitated by a fearful public without much pause for reflection. Although Nerlich *et al.* go on to argue that Dolly can be mobilized in both optimistic and pessimistic future scenarios and identify several discourses at work here, notably discourse of 'reason', 'fantasy', 'doom' 'hubris' (ibid.), they do not look closely at the links between these discourses and other social relations. The ways in which distribution of health care resources, the medicalization of fertility and pregnancy, access to essential services, agricultural practices, the treatment of children, the links between private capital and scientific research, the inadequacies of government regulation of global bioscience, become frames for these cloning discussions are not really considered. As Franklin argues with respect to Dolly the sheep clones and stories about them can be thought of as 'embodiments of shifting and uncertain relationalities' (2001: 3). Paraphrasing Franklin once more, this raises important questions:

> the connections that link animal genealogy to human futures through industrialization, redefining basic issues of health, subsistence and economy in ways that produce new forms of citizenship as well.
>
> (Franklin, 2001: 9)

Petersen finds similar concerns with identity and 'human nature' in his analysis of the Australian press coverage about cloning (2002). He is critical of the ways these issues become bound up in moral discourses, and the consequent lack of attention to the complexities of the social environment and its interactions with genes. However, he notes that press coverage of cloning involves discussion about the motives and interests of scientists that are not usually part of a news media that tends to portray scientists as heroes. Van Dijck concurs with these analyses, when she notes that, since the 1960s, 'two topoi have dominated popular fiction and non-fiction tales of genetic engineering: the subconscious desire to prolong human life, and the *Angst* over the loss of human identity and uniqueness' (Van Dijck, 1998: 184).

Cloning stories can be thought of as a way in which their writers negotiate these concerns and connections, sometimes deliberately deploying irony and exaggeration in order to stimulate further discussion, at other times caricaturing their opponents as fearful and irresponsible in order to underline the rationality of their own argument. Indeed, cloning stories are one area where the otherwise predominant discourse of market liberalism is actually being questioned. In these discourses risks are not bracketed or downplayed, but represented in technicolour. Desires for perfection and enhancement are considered in terms of exaggerated social divisions. The potential for the rich and famous to realize the human desire for perfection is questioned, albeit within a nihilistic framework where it is thought to be inevitable that these technologies will be developed and applied by an exotic minority.

Mass media discussion of designer babies in the British press at least, often has a similar format, painting risks in broad brush strokes, and failing to interrogate the complexities of the identities or technologies that genetic manipulation of the embryo might involve (Nerlich *et al.*, 2002). However, as with cloning, exaggerated risks are not simply produced by opponents of these types of developments. The term, designer baby, like references to Frankenstein or Brave New World, is often used by scientists and other proponents of new genetic technologies who are keen to ridicule their opponents and promote the familiar tropes of curing disease and unlocking natures' secrets (see also Mulkay, 1997; Kitzinger and Williams, 2004). Media discussion about designer babies also begins to explore the consequences of selecting foetuses with socially desirable but non-medical traits, and the termination of foetuses with trivial impairments.

There is some evidence to suggest that these frameworks are a product of the structures and values of the media industry. As Conrad and Markens have argued with respect to different styles of reporting about the so-called 'gay gene' in the United States and United Kingdom,

> news can be seen as reenacting beliefs for a community in addition to transmitting a message. Thus taking an optimistic frame about the 'gay gene' perhaps reasserts the US belief in the positive power of science, while the British framing reflects a deeper cultural distrust in science or a 'rhetoric of concern'.... Thus, the news framing is less about social views of genetics and homosexuality than it is about what each culture values.
>
> (Conrad and Markens, 2001: 393)

The ways in which journalists approach these issues also depend upon the structure of their relationships with national and international scientists and activists and the ways in which they relate to each other, their editors and political allies (ibid.). This involves different notions of citizenship and individual liberty, as well as scientific freedom, regulatory control and social divisions. At times, these frames can open up critical discussion, as discussed here. However, it is also important to note that at other times, as in the recent discussion of stem cell research, they can foreclose debate (Kitzinger and Williams, 2004).

Williams *et al.* (2003) describe this process in their analysis of the coverage in the British press around the Donaldson report (Chief Medical Officer's Expert Group, 2000), where therapeutic uses of stem cells was advocated. As Williams *et al.* argue, coverage was replete with images of stem cell scientists as pioneers (as suggested by proponents of research) or pirates (as suggested by opponents). They argue that although these images

> appear to be in fundamental opposition, they share an underlying logic. Both, in part, draw their power from a deeply racialized notion of civilization versus primitive barbarity, both leave the concept of 'progress' unquestioned.
>
> (Williams *et al.*, 2003: 810)

Williams *et al.* go on to argue that these kinds of tropes meant that there was a lack of attention, by proponents and critics of stem cell research alike, to the gap between the future cures and the reality of stem cell research. The wider social and political context of biomedicine, particularly limits on choice, the commodification of stem cell lines and invasive treatments on women who will supply the eggs and embryos required for stem cells to be harvested (ibid.) also tended to be ignored. Discussion of the potential benefits of embryonic stem cell research involved constructing patient identities based on innocence, suffering and hope:

> Hope is not identified as a human aspiration or emotion. Nor is there much discussion of the potential gap between wishful thinking and reality. Instead hope is presented as a basis for claim making and as an imperative to action ... To deny suffers hope... is [presented as] unnecessary and cruel.
>
> (Kitzinger and Williams, 2004: 15)

As the discussion in Chapter 3 illustrated, press releases and press conferences are important in shaping journalists' presentation of genetics news, and often give rise to an optimistic, technocratic model of progress. As Kitzinger and Williams argue, media reportage is predominantly a male narrative, largely produced by and for men. It is also 'event oriented', and often polarized, although personal accounts from patients are increasingly mobilized in 'hard' news formats to emphasize their human interest value (ibid.).

As Van Dijck explains, 'despite ardent insistence on professional divisions of labour, the "image" of genetics is produced simultaneously by scientists, journalists and public relations managers' (Van Dijck, 1998: 190). It is also important to note that journalists and their sources co-construct their readership and their predilections for certain stories and future scenarios as part of their work. Although this is based, in part, upon market research, it nevertheless involves considerable efforts in imagining readers' desires, interests and foibles, a process that inevitably reflects the interests, habits and priorities of journalists and their fellow storytellers.

Conclusion

These various types of future discourses construct the public, patients, scientists and technologies in particular ways that reflect the values and aspirations of their creators. The public are often castigated for their passivity, naivety and taste for the extreme, whereas patients are individualized on the one hand, or grouped together as hopeful, but miserable, unfortunates on the other. In much of the work on futures, humanity as a whole is given certain immutable desires, such as the quest for perfection and longevity. The more essentialized these identities become the more their authors retreat from the complex and multiple realities of people's existence. Scientists and doctors have more virile and active identities: seeking, curing and responding to need. Their intentions may be questioned, but rarely are the details of their working practices considered. Instead, the caricature of the mad scientists becomes a vehicle for morality tales about the misuse of science. Technology is a means through which human instincts are realized. The quest for perfection may be of concern to some, but it is cast as inevitable by others. The importance of progress is largely uncontested. Just as scientists' practices tend to be unexamined, so too do the processes of developing, manufacturing and marketing new technologies. Scientists', publics' and patients' identities are curiously fixed even as their authors purport to be engaging with an open future, or exploring the multiple, fractured identities of the postmodern age. Perhaps ironically, it is the mass media that seems to offer a more broad ranging, if controversial, discussion of the future of new technologies such as genetic enhancement and reproductive cloning, engaging with, rather than dismissing the economic and political context of professional practice, albeit in a format of exaggeration and hype.

Further reading

Ashcroft, R. (2003) 'American biofutures: ideology and utopia in the Fukuyama–Stock debate', *Journal of Medical Ethics*: 29:1, 59–62.

Brown, N., Rappert, B. and Webster, A. (eds) (2000) *Contested Futures: A Sociology of Prospective Techno-science*, Aldershot: Ashgate.

Petersen, A. (2002) 'Replicating our bodies, losing our selves: news media portrayals of human cloning in the wake of Dolly', *Body & Society*, 8:4, 71–90.

Van Dijck, J. (1998) *Imagenation: Popular Images of Genetics*, London: Macmillan.

Williams, C., Kitzinger, J. and Henderson, L. (2003) 'Envisaging the embryo in stem cell research: rhetorical strategies and media reporting of the ethical debates', *Sociology of Health and Illness*, 25:7, 793–814.

9 Conclusion

Introduction

> The more important task is to engage the essential ambivalence of artefacts in general. This requires us to give centre stage to our mundane experiences of technology, and to all the contradictions and tensions involved: technology is good and bad; it is enabling and it is oppressive; it works and it does not; and, as just part of all this, it does and does not have politics. These tensions are a significant manifestation of the competing discourses to which our experience of technology is subject, and within which we make sense of them. The very richness of this phenomenon suggests that it is insufficient to resolve the tensions by recourse to a quest for a definitive account of the actual character of a technology.
>
> (Woolgar and Cooper, 1999: 443)

Taken as a whole, this book presents something of a contradiction. On the one hand, I have outlined the diverse and contested discourses, experiences, and relationships associated with genetics and society. On the other hand, I am now supposed to offer some kind of overarching analysis of genetics and society. This means that this concluding chapter must steer away from grand analysis, while at the same time saying something meaningful about the extent of the diversity of the discourses, subject positions and relationships between human and non-human actors that have been discussed in the course of the book. How heterogeneous and flexible are the discourses around genetics and society? Are there any commonalities in the ways in which different social actors account for genetic technologies, diseases, and patients' and publics' relationships to them? What tensions about the risks and/or the benefits of genetics endure?

Conclusions also ought to say something about the strengths and weaknesses of the scholarship that has been surveyed in the course of the book. This requires yet more careful negotiation, as this scholarship is diverse and open to various interpretations in its own right. It should, however, be possible to respect this diversity, indeed applaud it, and at the same time identify some aspects of genetics and society that could be fruitfully explored in order to enhance the field. At the same time, it would be naïve to operate with the assumption that funding bodies will finance a great diversity of social research, given that there are very real restrictions on what is possible in this area.

Past, present and future

A central theme in this book has been the relationships between the past, present and future. I did not set out to trace how genetics and society have changed, but to look at the various stories that are told about their past, present and future. How diverse and flexible are these stories? What assumptions and tensions persist therein? What do they tell us about the relationships between genetics and society? Can we detect a growing scepticism about the projects of modernity, especially social progress and enlightenment? Do the actors in these stories, human and non-human, have clear identities? Are the boundaries between the social and the natural, knowledge and ideology and the individual and society breaking down?

In Chapter 2, I argued that there are a number of enduring themes in discourses about the relationships between eugenics and genetics, but these discourses are also flexible and heterogeneous. In contrast to the past, the individual is privileged in many discussions about genetics today, as are the complexities of genes. Yet, there remains a strong emphasis upon preventing deviance and disease through medical rather than social interventions. These aspects of genetics and society are nevertheless interpreted in a number of ways, by a range of different groups, to support various practices. Sometimes distinctions between the past and the present are challenged in arguments against one technology, but are deployed in arguments in support of another. This diversity reflects the flexible relationships and identities in the contemporary era. It also reflects the considerable levels of ambivalence about developments in genetics, especially their place in commerce and governance, and the multiplicity of actors that are involved in these processes.

Discourses of the future share some of these characteristics. A range of futures is apparent in the literature on genetics, variously stressing cures and/or risks. The individual is often privileged therein, as is the prevention of disease. These discourses are constructed by a range of social actors, and the ways in which the past, present and future are framed reflect their different aspirations, as well as the constraints placed upon them when producing their visions of the future. This means that particular notions of choice and social benefits are mobilized in different ways, depending upon the context.

A number of enduring themes are, however, apparent in these discourses of past and future. The benefits and risks of these new technologies are an important theme in all of the discussions of genetics and society. Social progress, the prevention of disease, and individual choice are lined up against discrimination and stigma, instrumentalization, and social control. Tensions are most profound when it comes to the relationship between the individual and society. The extent to which people can or should exercise choice as autonomous agents; the rights and responsibilities which come with individual choice, for both the person doing the choosing and the professionals charged with its steerage; and the social consequences of choices, for disabled people, parents of affected individuals and our future progeny – all of these issues are especially contentious. However, this focus upon individuals' choices and their consequences, seems to take attention away from professionals' and politicians' choices to develop and support particular genetic technologies. In many ways, these discourses close down discussions that they purport to be opening up, by constructing very narrow subject positions for consumers, patients, and publics, and by imbuing technologies with an inevitability, borne out of humanities' quest for improvement and perfection. In many instances, genes and diseases are presented as immutable objects, especially in policy documents, popular science and academic bioethics. Their materiality is simply assumed. Genes wait to be discovered, and although negative consequences may flow from their discovery, they are rarely considered to be active agents in their own right. Technologies too have an apparently limitless power to transform social relationships in these kinds of discourses. The overwhelming tendency to focus upon the impact of these technologies implies that they are produced and sustained by magical means. Somewhat ironically, it seems that the 'hype' around genetics in popular media accounts of new developments such as cloning, is one of the few discourses that actually opens up space for critical reflection of these issues. In these formats, professional practice and social exclusion comes under considerable scrutiny, in contrast to the prevailing tendency in much of bioethics to promote the benefits of liberal capitalism.

A range of social actors are critical of the ways in which boundaries between the past and the present are presented by the advocates of the new genetics, and of the post-human futures which have been promoted alongside them. However, alternative discourses do not necessarily challenge the foundations of modernity, but reassert them in an alternative form: progress here means equality; and enlightenment means an appreciation of the social as well as the biological causes of disease. Complex genes are mobilized at different points in these oppositional stories, but their role in exposing reductionism is fairly limited. It is only in a relatively small segment of the sociological literature on genetics that we see the boundaries between the social and the natural, knowledge and ideology, and humans and non-humans being deconstructed.

Patients, professionals and publics

The ways in which various subject positions are constructed in discourses about genetics and society is the second main theme of this book. Chapter 5 on 'Patients' and Chapter 7 on 'Publics' addressed these themes explicitly, but I have not produced a chapter about professionals. This speaks for the lack of literature on professional practice in this area, and the tendency to black box professionals' roles, alongside the genes, knowledge and technologies with which they work. Professionals are something of an absent present in the literature on genetics and society. This means that although a great deal of this book raises questions about their role in genetics and society, this forms a series of threads rather than a substantive topic in its own right.

In the course of writing, I have become much more conscious of the ways in which these actors are produced through the stories we tell about ourselves and others, rather than pre-existing positions which people occupy without much thought. Perhaps this reflects a newfound fluidity in contemporary identity politics. Or, it may be a just a newfound preoccupation with flexibility, which does not mean that identities were not flexible in the past as well. However, we should try to be aware of these complexities when analysing people's accounts of genetics and society.

The subject position of patient is particularly interesting in this regard. When constructed by health professionals, stories about patients are often a means by which to underline the benefits of technological advance, particularly when it comes to diagnosis and cure. Genes are the implicit bedrock of patient's identities and experiences. Finding genes and fixing them, at once constructs and erases the category of patient.

However, only certain kinds of patients seem to be a source of inspiration in this way. Much of the work of contemporary genetics stretches the notion of patient to include many people who have an element of genetic risk of illness in the future. Their stories seem to be of more interest than those of some other groups who are more likely to welcome the category of patient, particularly those who are socially excluded and marginalized from mainstream health services.

The category of patient is nevertheless contested in a number of respects, by social researchers keen to explore the multiple identities which people affected by genetic disease construct and enact in the course of their daily lives, and by other groups of disability and patient activists who variously seek to reject medical paternalism and assert their rights to be normal or normalized.

The same dynamics of reification and rejection can be seen when it comes to the category of public. Despite an apparent range of tools and strategies to engage the public in discussions about genetics and society, and a newfound emphasis upon dialogue with multiple publics rather than the education of an ignorant mass, a number of harder notions of what the public is, and where its qualities are wanting, seem to prevail. Publics continue to be framed as lacking knowledge, trust or impetus. Experts, on the other hand, have proliferated. This expertise may be contested and contingent, but the public seems to be many people's favourite 'bête noire'. Those who seek an authentic band of citizens who might exercise democratic control of sciences and technologies like genetics might create this version of the public in their own scholarship, but it does not seem to have much resonance outside the policy and academic networks for whom it is produced.

Professionals, or experts, are scattered throughout discussions of genetics and society rather than problematized in their own right. Yet, their ability to create their own identity discourses is unparalleled. There are multiple fora in which professionals can express their ambivalence about the social consequences of work involving genetics. These spaces of professional dialogue are probably not as new as we might think, but they have taken on a newfound significance in discussions about the risk society. Professionals' self-conscious positioning as ethical beings affords them an element of flexibility that other more marginalized groups seek but do not necessarily achieve because their access to discourse production is more constrained. At the same time, professional, like patient and public, is but one form of identity, and people can shift between and all of these identities in discourse and practice. Professionals must also contend with other groups who challenge and translate their discourses and practices, so that their claims to ethics and enlightenment are invariably contested. Various divisions also exist between professionals in terms of their disciplinary and institutional commitments and the ways in which they intersect with their other familial and personal identities. This means that their ethical discourses are always partial and contingent upon the context in which they are articulated.

Knowledge, practice and things

The third and final theme in this book concerns the social construction of genetic knowledge, the social and cultural contexts of laboratory, clinical and governance practices, and the place of genes in the story of genetics and society. Chapter 3 explicitly addresses the social and material actors involved in the processes of gene discovery, and the ways in which these come to be represented in popular formats such as the institutional press release. Genes are complicated things. The processes of identifying genes involve a dense network of associations between professionals, patients and the physical substances that they donate. On a larger scale, the commercial, institutional and public contexts of genetic science and medicine also shape the process of discovery and how it comes to be represented. Genes are, however, far from stable entities, and their role in disease is unclear in many respects. Definitions of disease and of the genetic factors involved therein are mutually constitutive, now as in the past. They are shaped by the diagnostic techniques and treatments of the present, as well as assumptions and hypotheses generated in the past. Ideas about diseases and genes are unstable and their relationships are unpredictable. These contingent and provisional aspects of genes are not unique to the contemporary era, but an intrinsic part of scientific enquiry. However, much of this complexity is deleted in the politics of genetics writ large.

Genes and other biochemical or biological entities nevertheless form an important part of the story of how particular technologies are developed and applied. Materiality shapes the process of technological design, placing limits upon what is possible, and how these limitations come to be categorized and perceived. Genes and other material entities also become a part of professionals' commitments to particular procedures and modes of operation. Certain research groups and institutions come to have a stake in searching for particular markers or mutations, as they have built up expertise in that area. Genes and other entities may attain biovalue, through patenting for example. This shapes the ways in which the technologies with which they are associated are translated into other clinical and institutional domains. However, the status of these genes as meaningful and/or financially valuable entities is also contested by other competing groups of researchers and clinicians, and increasingly patients themselves. At times this involves appeals to their fundamental role in the biological body: their status as discoveries, rather than creations or inventions of the research process. Such a discourse emphasizes their mundane, natural qualities. At other times they can become important aspects of people's identities – an important part of the patient that they have become. This places emphasis upon the patients' ownership of their genes, rather than the scientists or clinicians with an interest in their condition.

However, genes are also frustratingly difficult to find in many of the discourses about the social aspects of genetics. Complex genes seem to reside in laboratories, and they are often translated into facts of nature beyond the laboratory walls. Bringing their contingency back into the stories of genetics and society is an uphill struggle. Some professionals will share their experiences of genetic complexity with social researchers and affected individuals in their efforts to account for their practice. People affected by genetic disorders often engage with the complexities of genes as they negotiate the meaning of disease. A range of scientific and critical commentators might mobilize genetic complexity in their arguments against the 'hype' of genetic reductionism and determinacy that surrounds high profile projects such as the Human Genome Project. These discourses are nevertheless overshadowed by a range of countervailing tendencies to black box genes and their complexities for public consumption. This is especially true when it comes to arguments in favour of new genetic diagnostic technologies and associated efforts to cure or prevent genetic disease.

Some of these processes are highlighted in Chapter 4 on reproductive genetic technologies and Chapter 6 on biobank research. The discourse of choice dominates much of the discussion of the social aspects of these areas of genetics, acting as a conduit for dialogue among a diverse range of stakeholders. However, this discourse masks many of the institutional and bureaucratic actors who engender and support practices such as genetic screening or databanking. The development of these technologies and their governance go hand in hand, so much so that the genetic knowledge that comes forth from their design is the product of multiple relationships between a range of close and distant actors. Despite the apparent impenetrability of genetic knowledge in the discourses of promise and progress around genetics, it is both provisional and contingent, subject to interpretation and reinterpretation by all of these actors, including the patients and donors from whom, and for whom, it is apparently conceived. This is both an outcome and a reflection of the variety of groups, individuals, entities and practices that make up genetic research in these areas. Flexible governance can foster flexible knowledge, and vice versa.

Researching genetics and society

I began this book by querying social researchers' apparent fascination with new and transformative aspects of genetics, as opposed to its not so new, or mundane aspects. I deliberately constructed the analysis in such a way as to problematize notions of the new and to explore several genetic technologies and practices that are fairly established, notably the identification of genes for disease, and reproductive screening. I was able to draw on a considerable number of more ethnographic studies of laboratory and clinical practice, and to build my own analysis of discourse, governance, and professional practice into the story of the new and the not so new aspects of genetics. However, I also noted a preponderance of research into patients' experiences and publics' perceptions of genetics. I expressed frustration about the narrow focus upon the impact of technology in much of this work, as opposed to the social conditions through which technologies are designed, and the multiple perspectives and relationships which people go on to have with them. I noted that social researchers who are oriented towards improving clinical practice or democratic consultation processes must shape their analyses according to the needs of their commissioners. Although this can be valuable in terms of improving the processes of implementing particular technologies, it does little to address the question of whether or not these technologies should be developed in the first place.

This does not, however, mean that I am proposing that social researchers should turn their attentions to designing better technologies. Surely, this is the job of scientists and clinicians, rather than the people who study their practice. I do, nevertheless, want to raise the question of how social researchers account for their work and their relationships to funding bodies, practitioners and so-called user groups. This involves some awkward questions about the concentration of so much social research on new areas of science such as genetics. Many researchers do not have much choice about which funding sources they will pursue, given the precarious nature of their employment. However, the predominant focus upon people's experiences of the impact and consequences of sciences and technologies, like genetics, is less than satisfactory. Opening up these issues to more critical scrutiny is a difficult task, but it need not involve regular pronouncements about what is acceptable and what is not, or a close involvement with policing the production and application of genetic knowledge and technologies.

There is much more scope for social scientists' involvement in open and critical dialogue about the politics of contemporary genetic knowledge and technologies in the local contexts in which it is being produced. The current emphasis upon interdisciplinarity is both a help and a hindrance in this regard. Although this can generate fruitful alliances between social scientists and the people whose experiences and practices they wish to understand, there is no denying that they do not come to these relationships on an equal footing. As anyone who has tried to interview a clinician or a scientist will verify, it is a very different experience from interviewing patients or members of the public. This is largely because clinicians and scientists tend to consider their work and their interpretations of that work as more robust, objective and socially useful than the work of many of their colleagues in the social sciences. In contrast, so-called lay people often struggle to find answers to social researchers' questions because they find them intimidating. This is not necessarily because they hold their interviewers in particularly high esteem, but because the interview is a rather odd and unsettling form of conversation where they must translate their experiences to suit the researchers' needs. Clinicians and scientists have a variety of techniques for circumventing this type of relationship with social researchers, not least the dismissal of their questions as irrelevant or obtuse.

Persistence and patience can, however, pay off, as a number of fascinating ethnographic studies of laboratory and clinical practice have demonstrated (Batchelor *et al.*, 1996; Franklin, 1997; Fujimura, 1997; Rapp, 2000). Research which aims to explore a field or an area of practice, as opposed to the views of a particular group or the social factors influencing certain perceptions, allows for much more reflexive and creative analyses of social action. This type of work is thoroughly grounded in an understanding of practice, but it is far from naïve realism, as the complexities of practice cannot be understood without a sound theoretical framework. Actor network and social world theories, as well as broader analyses of materiality and social action are important in this regard (see Fujimura, 1997; Latour, 2003). All of these approaches bring the material back into the story of science and technology.

This type of approach can also be valuable without the laboratory and the clinic, as a way of understanding the complexities of people's experiences of genetic disease, or involvement in patient groups, and the governance of genetics more broadly. Genetic knowledge and the research and technologies with which it is associated mean many things to different people. They can be both mundane and unusual, helpful and oppressive. In order to understand these rich and dynamic processes we must move beyond the narrow categories of patient or lay expert, to look at genetics in the wider context of people's lives. We must also understand that genetic knowledge and technologies are often at the background of people's life worlds, lacking relevancy and saliency for the most part, except when it comes to key life events such as pregnancy or serious illness. This suggests that we should turn our attention to other more mundane aspects of people's engagement with science and technology as well, rather than focusing upon how the next revolutionary health technology may, or may not, transform their sense of self.

The area which is probably most in need of critical research is, however, governance. An ethnographic approach to governance is difficult to negotiate, despite the burgeoning rhetoric of transparency and accountability. Ethics committees and policy-making bodies remain largely closed to critical scrutiny, as do the ways in which professionals negotiate ethics in their daily work. However, Jasanoff (1990), Mulkay (1997), and Kelly (2003) have given important insights into the policy-making process. They have considered the negotiation of boundaries between and around experts, publics and controversial entities such as embryos, stressing the construction of discourses of consensus and publics therein. The operation of these kinds of policy bodies as 'border guards' (Kelly, 2003: 358) of scientific expertise and autonomy is particularly interesting. In the United Kingdom, other researchers have also begun to study the practices of bodies like the Human Genetic Commission, in an effort to understand these processes. It may also be the case that exploring these aspects of genetic governance will turn out to an important point of access to the study of governance more generally.

Exploring genetics and society need not involve the perpetuation of common tropes of individual choice, social progress and transformative technologies. Social research can reflect upon the place of these kinds of discourses, at the same time as it unpacks the relationships between the people and things that underpin them. This opens, rather than closes, dialogue about the development of genetic technologies and their place in social life. I hope that this book has contributed to these processes of analysis, reflection and debate.

Glossary

Aetiology   Refers to the cause of a disease.

Age-related aneuploidies   Refers to chromosomal abnormalities resulting from increased maternal age.

Alpha fetoprotein   Alpha fetoprotein is present in pregnant women's blood. High levels of apha fetoprotein are associated with foetal abnormality. Women who have high levels of alpha fetoprotein between 16 and 18 weeks of pregnancy will be offered amniocentesis to measure alpha fetoprotein levels in the amniotic fluid. High levels may indicate that the foetus has a neural tube defect. When low levels of alpha fetoprotein occur alongside high levels of other biochemical markers in the mother's blood, the foetus might have Down's syndrome. Other factors also influence the level of alpha fetoprotein in a pregnant woman, including the length of the pregnancy.

Amniocentesis   Amniocentesis is used to detect abnormalities in a foetus. A doctor inserts a needle through the pregnant woman's abdomen and collects a sample of amniotic fluid which surrounds the foetus in the womb. Amniocentesis is usually performed between 15 and 17 weeks of pregnancy. There is a risk of miscarriage which is variously estimated at between 0.5 and 2 per cent.

Antenatal screening   Antenatal screening, sometimes also known as prenatal screening, refers to tests that are offered to a defined population of pregnant women, usually in the early stages of pregnancy, to detect foetal abnormalities. Women identified as having higher risk will then be offered follow-up testing, such as amniocentesis. This can be contrasted with antenatal testing, which is offered to women whose foetuses are already known to be at a high risk of a particular genetic disorder. Examples of antenatal screening include Down's syndrome screening, currently offered to women over the age of 35 in the United Kingdom, but soon to be extended to all pregnant women.

Biochemical markers   Alpha fetoprotein is one example of a biochemical marker which can be found in pregnant women's blood. Markers are chemical elements of pregnant women's blood, high or low levels of which are known to be associated with particular foetal abnormalities.

BRCA1 *BRCA1* is a gene that is involved in some forms of hereditary breast and ovarian cancer.

Celera Inc. This company was formed by Craig Venter in 1993. Celera aimed to sequence the interesting parts of the human genome in three years, using a technique known as whole genome shotgun sequencing. This technique was less precise than the methods used by the Human Genome Project (HGP), and less expensive. Celera also planned to patent their results and set up a database to which genetic researchers could subscribe. Celera and the HGP published their draft results at the same time in different journals, and Francis Collins the director of the HGP stood alongside Craig Venter at the White House press conference to mark the occasion.

Chorionic villus sampling CVS is used to detect abnormalities in the foetus, usually between 10 and 12 weeks of pregnancy. A sample of the chorionic villi is taken from the placenta, through the cervix or the abdominal wall. Chorionic villi are small projections that make up part of the placenta, extending into the walls of the uterus, allowing the exchange of oxygen, nutrients and waste materials between mother and foetus. CVS is sometimes favoured over amniocentesis because it can be performed earlier in the pregnancy.

Chromosomal abnormalities Chromosomes are coils of DNA which are contained within the nucleus of every cell in the body. People usually have 23 pairs of chromosomes. Chromosomal abnormalities affect the size, number or arrangements of parts of chromosomes. Down's syndrome occurs because of an extra chromosome, usually number 21.

Clinical genetics Clinical genetics or medical genetics involves doctors in the study, identification and treatment of genetic diseases.

Cloning Cloning is an imprecise term, which usually refers to the introduction of genetic material into the nucleus of an egg through artificial means in order to produce a genetic copy of a particular organism. Dolly the sheep is the most famous clone. She was created when scientists fused a mammary gland cell from a dead sheep with an enucleated egg (an egg from which the nucleus had been removed).

Coeliac disease Coeliac disease is an inherited intolerance to gluten, a protein found in wheat and rye, which causes changes in the intestine that result in problems with digesting and absorbing foods.

Congenital Congenital means from birth, and refers to abnormalities, for example congenital blindness.

Cystic fibrosis Cystic fibrosis is a genetic disease, inherited in a Mendelian recessive pattern. It usually becomes apparent in early childhood, characteristically involving a build-up of mucous in the lungs and problems with digestion, but it can affect all of the organs in the body to varying degrees.

DNA Deoxyribonucleic acid is the body's genetic material – the main element of the chromosomes of all living organisms. It takes the form of a double helix, resembling a spiral staircase. DNA is self-replicating and transmits hereditary characteristics. DNA contains genes which code for the production of particular proteins.

Duchenne Muscular Dystrophy   An X-linked recessive disease (i.e. females are carriers), causing weakness and wasting of muscles.

Exocrine glands   These glands release their products onto the free surface of the skin or onto the free surface of the open cavities of the body such as the digestive, respiratory or reproductive tracts, rather than the blood.

Fanconi Anaemia   Fanconi Anaemia is a rare disorder found in children that involves the blood and bone marrow. The symptoms include severe aplastic anaemia, hypoplasia of the bone marrow, and patchy discoloration of the skin. This is an autosomal recessive condition, affected children usually develop severe aplastic anaemia by age 8–9 years.

Genotype   The genetic make-up of an organism.

Germline gene therapy   Germline gene therapy is aimed at correcting defective genes. Unlike somatic gene therapy, which would affect only the target cells of the individual being treated, germline therapy would have permanent hereditary consequences.

Human Genome Project   The Human Genome Project (1990–2003) sequenced the entire human genome and identified all of the genes in human DNA. The information is stored in databases with the aim of developing better means of identifying and treating genetic disease.

Huntington's disease   Huntington's disease (HD) results from the degeneration of brain cells, called neurons, in certain areas of the brain. This degeneration causes uncontrolled movements, loss of intellectual faculties and emotional disturbance. HD is a familial disease, passed from parent to child through a mutation in the normal gene. Each child of an HD parent has a 50–50 chance of inheriting the HD gene.

Hypercholesterolaemia   Familial hypercholesterolaemia is a rare inherited disease of metabolism. The normal process that removes cholesterol particles from the blood stream does not work in patients with this disease. It causes cholesterol to build-up in the arteries and leads to hardening of the arteries (atherosclerosis).

In vitro fertilization (IVF)   IVF is a method of assisted reproduction in which the man's sperm and the woman's egg are combined in a laboratory dish, where fertilization occurs. The resulting embryo is then transferred to the uterus.

Inhibin-A   A marker for Down's syndrome in pregnancy.

Mendelian recessive disorder   So-called autosomal recessive disorders are caused by an error or mutation in a single unit of genetic information. An autosomal disorder that is recessive can be expressed in a person only if both copies of the gene are altered. When both parents are carriers of the same recessive gene, there is a 25 per cent risk with each pregnancy that the child will receive both recessive genes and be affected with the disorder.

Multifactorial condition   A condition that is caused by the interaction of genetic factors and the environment.

Neural tube defects   Birth defects of the baby's brain (anencephaly) or spine (spina bifida).

Nuchal translucency thickness   An ultrasound measurement of the fluid accumulation, or nuchal translucency, in the neck of foetuses that causes abnormal swelling or enlargement – an indicator of a chromosomal defect.

Pharmacogenomics   Pharmacogenomics is the study of how an individual's genetic inheritance affects the body's response to drugs.

Phenotype   The outward, physical manifestation of the organism.

Preimplantation genetic diagnosis   Preimplantation genetic diagnosis (PGD) is a technique that can be used during in vitro fertilization (IVF) procedures to test embryos for genetic disorders prior to their transfer to the uterus.

Presymptomatic test   Presymptomatic testing is a method for identifying persons with genes that can cause disease before the symptoms appear.

PXE   Pseudoxanthoma elasticum is an inherited disorder that affects tissue in some parts of the body, causing calcium and other minerals to be deposited in the tissue, affecting the skin, eyes, cardiovascular system and gastrointestinal system.

Sickle-cell disease   Sickle cell disease is an inherited blood disorder that affects red blood cells. People with sickle cell disease have red blood cells that contain mostly haemoglobin S, an abnormal type of haemoglobin. Sometimes these become sickle shaped and have difficulty passing through small blood vessels, blocking blood flow and damaging tissue.

Single nucleotide polymorphisms (SNPs)   Common DNA sequence variations among individuals.

Somatic gene therapy   Aims to replace defective genes with normal versions to prevent or treat disease.

Steatorrhoea   Steatorrhoea is the name used to describe the condition where there is an increased amount of fat passed via the bowel, producing stools that are pale, greasy and offensive. This is due to malabsorption of fat either because of pancreatic disease or small intestinal disease such as Coeliac disease.

Stem cells   Stem cells are different from other types of cells because they are unspecialized cells that renew themselves for long periods through cell division. Under certain conditions, they can be induced to become cells with special functions such as the beating cells of the heart muscle. Scientists work with two kinds of stem cells from animals and humans: embryonic stem cells and adult stem cells, which have different functions and characteristics.

Werdnig-Hoffman's syndrome   A form of spinal muscular atrophy that leads to degeneration of the spinal column and progressive loss of control of muscle movements. The disease is inherited in a recessive pattern and the child dies within the first two years.

Notes

1 Introduction

1 See http://www.york.ac.uk/res/iht/
2 See http://www.wellcome.ac.uk/en/1/mismis.html
3 Cunningham-Burley, S., Amos, A. (Principal Investigators) and Kerr, A. (Research Fellow): 'The Social and Cultural Impact of the New Genetics', Public Health Sciences, University of Edinburgh, funded by the ESRC Research Programme on Risk and Human Behaviour, 1 November 1994 to 31 July 1997; and Kerr, A., Cunningham-Burley, S. (Principal Investigators) and Tutton, R. (Research Fellow): 'Transformations in Genetic Subjecthood' (TIGS), Department of Sociology, University of York and Public Health Sciences, University of Edinburgh funded by the ESRC Innovative Health Technologies Programme, 1 April 2002 to 31 March 2004 http://www.york.ac.uk/res/tigs/ Reference Number: L218252059.
4 Kerr, A. (Principal Investigator) 'A history of cystic fibrosis: definition and diagnosis 1938 – the present', Science Studies Unit, University of Edinburgh and Department of Sociology, University of York, funded by The Wellcome Trust, History of Medicine Fellowship, 1997–2002. Grant Number: 050419.

3 Discovery

1 Cf. note 3, TIGS project.
2 Cf. note 4.

6 Biobanks

1 Cf. note 3, TIGS project.

7 Publics

1 Cf. note 3, TIGS project.

Bibliography

Abraham, J. and Lewis, G. (2002) 'Citizenship, medical expertise and the capitalist regulatory state in Europe', *Sociology*, 31:1, 67–88.

Albert, B. (1999) 'If you tolerate this your children will be next', *Health Matters*, 36, Spring. Available at <http://www.healthmatters.org.uk/stories/albert.html> (accessed 29 October 2003).

Allen, G. (1983) 'The misuse of biological hierarchies: the American eugenics movement, 1900–1940', *History and Philosophy of the Life Sciences*, 5:2, 105–28.

ALSPAC Advisory and Executive Management Structures. Available at <http://www.alspac.bris.ac.uk/ALSPACext/MainProtocol/Appendix1.htm> (accessed 22 December 2003).

Anderson, R. (1999) 'Information technology in medical practice: safety and privacy lessons from the United Kingdom', *Medical Journal of Australia*, 170:4, 181–4, referenced in Churches, T. (2003) 'A proposed architecture and method of operation for improving the protection of privacy and confidentiality in disease registers', *BMC Medical Research Methodology*, 3:1, 1.

Anderton, J., Effert, H. and Lai, M. (1989) 'Ideology in the clinical context: chronic illness ethnicity and the discourse of normalisation', *Sociology of Health and Illness*, 11:3(Sep.) 253–78.

Anonymous (1979) 'Cystic fibrosis in adults', *British Medical Journal*, 2: 626.

—— (2001) 'Perfect?', *The Economist*, 11 April.

Antonellis, A., Ellsworth, R., Sambuughin, N., Puls, I., Abel, A., Lee-Lin, S.-Q., Jordanova, A., Kremensky, I., Christodoulou, K. and Middleton, L.T. (2003) 'Glycyl tRNA Synthetase Mutations in Charcot-Marie-Tooth Disease Type 2D and Distal Spinal Muscular Atrophy Type V', *American Journal of Human Genetics*, 72:5, 1293–9.

Ashcroft, R. (2003) 'American biofutures: ideology and utopia in the Fukuyama-Stock debate', *Journal of Medical Ethics*, 29:1, 59–62.

Atkin, K., Ahmad, W. and Anionwu, E., (1998) 'Screening and counselling for sickle cell disorders and thalassaemia: the experience of parents and health professionals', *Social Science and Medicine*, 47:11, 1639–51.

Bailey, R. (1996) 'Prenatal testing and the prevention of impairment: a woman's right to choose?', in J. Morris (ed.) *Encounters with Strangers: Feminism and Disability*, London: Women's Press, 143–67.

Balmer, B. (1996) 'Managing mapping of the Human Genome Project', *Social Studies of Science*, 26: 531–73.

Barbero, G. and Sibinga, M. (1959) 'The electrolyte abnormality in cystic fibrosis of the pancreas', *Pediatric Clinics of North America*, 6: 221–40.

Barbour, V. (2003) 'UK Biobank: a project in search of a protocol?', *The Lancet*, 361: 1734–8.

Batchelor, C., Parsons, E. and Atkinson, P. (1996) 'The career of a medical discovery', *Qualitative Health Research*, 6: 224–55.

Beaudry, P. (1987) 'Cystic fibrosis – clinical viewpoint – a disease that doesn't make sense', *Progress in Clinical and Biological Research*, 254: 1–5.

Beck, U. (1993) *Die Erfindung des Politischen*; trans. Mark Ritter (1997) *The Reinvention of Politics: Rethinking Modernity in the Global Social Order*, Cambridge: Polity Press.

—— (1995) *Ecological Politics in an Age Of Risk*, Cambridge: Polity Press.

Berg, K. (2001) 'DNA sampling and banking in clinical genetics and genetic research', *New Genetics and Society*, 20:1, 59–68.

Beskow, L., Burke, W., Merz, J., Barr, P., Terry, S., Penchaszadeh, V., Gostin, L., Gwinn, M. and Khoury, M. (2001) 'Informed consent for population-based research involving genetics', *Journal of the American Medical Association*, 286:18, 2315–21.

Billings, P. (2000) 'Homecooked Eugenic', *GeneLetter*, 1:1 February.

Bindra, R., Heath, V., Liao, A., Spencer, K. and Nicolaides, K. (2002) 'One-stop clinic for assessment of risk for Trisomy 21 at 11–14 weeks: a prospective study of 15,030 pregnancies', *Ultrasound in Obstetrics and Gynecology*, 20: 219–25.

Black, E. (2003) 'We must keep eugenics away from genetics', *Newsday*, 15 October, p. A.31.

Bobrow, M. and Thomas, S. (2001) 'Patents in a genetic age', *Nature*, 409:6822, 763–4.

Bodmer, W. and Mackie, R. (1995) *The Book of Man: The Quest to Discover Our Genetic Heritage,* London, Acabus.

Boehringer, C. (1968) *Das Medizinische Prisma, 4, Cystische Fibrose, von Guido Fanconi.*

Bonnefort, J., Thuillier, L., Gigarel, N., Rochette, C., Briard, M. and Munnich, A. (1997) 'Prenatal diagnosis of cystic fibrosis', *Pediatric Pulmonology*, Supplement, 16:63–4.

Bourdieu, P. (1990) *In Other Words. Essays towards a Reflexive Sociology.* Collected and translated by Matthew Adamson, Cambridge: Polity.

Braude, P., Pickering, S., Flinter, F. and Mackie Ogilvie, C. (2002) 'Preimplantation genetic diagnosis', *Nature Review Genetics*, 3: 941–53.

Brock, D. (2002) 'Human cloning and our sense of self', *Science*, 296:5566, 314–6.

Brown, N., Rappert, B. and Webster, A. (eds) (2000) *Contested Futures: A Sociology of Prospective Techno-science*, Aldershot: Ashgate.

Brunger, F. and Lippman, A. (1995) 'Resistance and adherence to the norms of genetic counseling', *Journal of Genetic Counselling*, 4:3, 151.

Bury, M. (1982) 'Chronic illness as biographical disruption', *Sociology of Health and Illness*, 4:2, 167–82.

—— (2001) 'Illness narratives: facts or fiction?', *Sociology of Health and Illness*, 23:3, 263–85.

Busby, H. (2004) 'Blood donation for genetic research: what can we learn from donors' narratives?', in R. Tutton and O. Corrigan (eds) *Genetic Databases: Socio-ethical Issues in the Collection and Use of DNA*, London: Routledge.

Cambrosio, A., Limoges, C. and Pronovost, D. (1990) 'Representing biotechnology: an ethnography of Quebec science policy', *Social Studies of Science*, 20:2, 195–227.

Caplan, A., McGee, G. and Magnus, D. (1999) 'What is immoral about eugenics?', *British Medical Journal*, 319: 1284.

Caulfield, T., Upshur, R. and Daar, A. (2003) 'DNA databanks and consent: a suggested policy option involving an authorization model', *BMC Medical Ethics*, 4:1.

Caygill, H. (2003) *The Making of the Modern Body*, Theory, Culture and Society Series, London: Sage.

Chakravarti, A. and Little, P. (2003) 'Nature, nurture and human disease', *Nature*, 421: 412–4.

Chapman, E. (2002) 'The social and ethical implications of changing medical technologies: the views of people living with genetic conditions', *Journal of Health Psychology*, 7:2, 195–206.

Chapple, J. (1992) 'Genetic screening: brave New World or the boys from Brazil?', *British Journal of Hospital Medicine*, 47:7, 487–9.

Charmaz, K. (1983) 'Loss of self: a fundamental form of suffering in the chronically ill', *Sociology of Health and Illness*, 5:2, 168–94.

Chiapello, E. and Fairclough, N. (2002) 'Understanding the new management ideology: a transdisciplinary contribution from critical discourse analysis and new sociology of capitalism', *Discourse & Society*, 13:2, 185–208.

Chief Medical Officer's Expert Group (2000) *Stem Cell Research: Medical Progress with Responsibility*, London: Department of Health.

Christian Medical Fellowship (2001) *Genetics and Human Behaviour: The Ethical Context.* Available at <http://www.cmf.org.uk/> Then select: Ethics <Submissions to Government Committees> Genetics and Human Behaviour (accessed 3 November 2003).

Chrysanthou, M. (2002) 'Transparency and selfhood: utopia and the informed body', *Social Science and Medicine*, 54: 469–79.

Clarke, A. (1991) 'Is non-directive genetic counselling possible?', *The Lancet*, 338: 998–1000.

Collins, H. and Evans, R. (2002) 'The third wave of science studies: studies of expertise and experience', *Social Studies of Science*, 32: 235–96.

Conrad, P. (1999) 'A mirage of genes', *Sociology of Health and Illness*, 21:2, 228–39.

—— and Weinberg, D. (1996) 'Has the gene for alcoholism been discovered three times since 1980?', *Perspectives On Social Problems*, 8: 3–25.

—— and Markens, S. (2001) 'Constructing the "gay gene" in the news: optimism and skepticism in the US and British press', *Health*, 5:3, 373–400.

Council of Europe (1997) *Convention for the Protection of Human Rights and Dignity of the Human Being with regard to the Application of Biology and Medicine: Convention on Human Rights and Biomedicine*, ETS no. 164., Oviedo, 4 April. Available at <http://conventions.coe.int/treaty/en/Treaties/Html/164.htm> (accessed 12 January 2004).

Council of Europe Committee of Ministers (1997) *Recommendation No R (97) 5 of the Committee of Ministers to Member States on the Protection of Medical Data*. Available at <http://cm.coe.int/ta/rec/1997/97r5.html> (accessed 18 December 2003).

Cowen, L., Corey, M., Keenan, N., Simmons, R., Arndt, E. and Levison, H. (1985) 'Family adaptation and psychosocial adjustment to cystic fibrosis in the preschool child', *Social Science and Medicine*, 20:6, 553–60.

Cox, S. and McKellin, W. (1999) 'There's this thing in our family: predictive testing and the construction of risk for Huntington's Disease', in P. Conrad and P. Gabe (eds) *Sociological Perspectives on the New Genetics*, Oxford: Blackwell Publishers, 622–46.

Coyne, I. (1997) 'Chronic illness: the importance of support for families caring for a child with cystic fibrosis', *Journal of Clinical Nursing*, 6: 121–9.

Cragg Ross Dawson (2000) *Public Perceptions of the Collection of Human Biological Samples: summary report*, London: Wellcome Trust; Medical Research Council.

Cuckle, H. (2002) 'Growing complexity in the choice of Down's Syndrome screening policy', *Ultrasound in Obstetrics and Gynecology*, 19: 323–6.

Cunningham-Burley, S. and Kerr, A. (1999) 'Defining the "social": towards an understanding of scientific and medical discourses on the social aspects of the new human genetics', *Sociology of Health and Illness*, 21:5, 647–68.

Cyranoski, D. (2000) 'Singapore to create nationwide disease database', *Nature*, 407:6807, 935.

Davies, K. (1990) 'The search for the cystic fibrosis gene', *CF News*, Dec/Jan: 10–13.

Davies, P. (1991) 'Cystic fibrosis from bench to bedside', *New England Journal of Medicine*, 325: 575–7.

——, Drumm, M. and Konstan, M. (1996) 'Cystic fibrosis', *American Journal of Respiratory and Critical Care Medicine*, 154: 1229–56.

Davison, A., Barns, I. and Schibeci, R. (1997) 'Problematic publics: a critical review of surveys of public attitudes to biotechnology', *Science, Technology and Human Values*, 22:3, 317–48.

Department of Health (2003a) *Our Inheritance, Our Future: Realizing the Potential of Genetics in the NHS*, Norwich: HMSO.

—— (2003b; draft) *Research Governance Framework for Health and Social Care*, Department of Health. Available at <http://www.doh.gov.uk/research/documents/rd3/rgf2ndeditionv22300403.doc> (accessed 5 November 2003).

Dodge, J. and Ryley, H. (1982) 'Screening for cystic fibrosis', *Archives of Disease in Childhood*, 57:10, 774–80.

——, Morison, S., Lewis, P., Coles, E., Geddes, S., Russell, G., *et al.* (1997) 'Incidence, population and survival of CF in the UK 1968-95', *Archives of Disease in Childhood*, 77: 493–6.

Dreidger, D. (1989) *The Last Civil Rights Movement*, London: Hurst & Co.

Dunkerley, D. and Glasner, P. (1998) 'Empowering the public? Citizens' juries and the new genetic technologies', *Critical Public Health*, 8: 181–92.

Durant, J. and Hansen, A. (1995) 'The role of the media', in W. Kennet (ed.) *Parliaments and Screening. A conference on the Ethical and Social Problems Arising from Testing and Screening for HIV and AIDS. The role of Parliaments and the Media. Conference Report and Studies of the Handling of Bioethics in the Twelve National Parliaments of the European Union*, London: John Libby Eurotext.

Einsiedel, E. (2002) 'Assessing a controversial medical technology: Canadian public consultations on xenotransplantation', *Public Understanding of Science*, 11:4, 315–31.

Eliasoph, N. (1998) *Avoiding Politics: How Americans Produce Apathy in Everyday Life*, Cambridge: Cambridge University Press.

Engelhardt, H. (2002) 'Germline engineering: the moral challenges', *American Journal of Medical Genetics*, 108: 169–75.

Evans, G. and Durant, J. (1995) 'The relationship between knowledge and attitudes in the public understanding of science in Britain', *Public Understanding of Science*, 4: 57–74.

Ewbank, J. (1998) 'Problems of germline therapy', *Nature*, 392, 66–77, 16 April 1998, 645.

Fears, R. and Poste, G. (1999) 'Building population genetics using the UK NHS', *Science*, 284: 267–8.

Ferguson, M., Gartner, A. and Lipsky, D. (2000) 'The experience of disability in families: a synthesis of research and parent narratives', in E. Parens and A. Asch (eds), *Prenatal Testing and Disability Rights*, Washington, DC: Georgetown University Press, 72–94.

Finkler, K. (2000) *Experiencing the New Genetics: Family and Kinship on the Medical Frontier*, Philadelphia, PA: University of Pennsylvania Press.

——, Skrzynia, C. and Evans, J. (2003) 'The new genetics and its consequences for family, kinship, medicine and medical genetics', *Social Science and Medicine*, 57: 403–12.

Fleischer, M. (2001) 'Patent thyself', *The American Lawyer*, 21 June.

Franklin, S. (1997) *Embodied Progress: A Cultural Account of Assisted Conception*, London: Routledge.

—— (2001) 'Culturing biology: cell lines for the second millennium', *Health*, 5:3, 335–54.

—— and Roberts, C. (2001) 'The social life of the embryo', paper presented at 'Ethnographies of the Centre', Lancaster University. Available at <http://www.comp.lancs.ac.uk/sociology/iht/eofcpaper.htm> (accessed 12 January 2004).

Fujimura, J. (1997) 'The practices of producing meaning in bioinformatics', *Sociology of the Sciences*, 21: 49–88.

—— (1998) 'The molecular bandwagon in cancer research: where social worlds meet', *Social Problems*, 35: 261–83.

Fukuyama, F. (2002) *Our Posthuman Future: Consequences of the Biotechnology Revolution*, New York: Picador.

General Medical Council (2000) *Confidentiality: Protecting and Providing Information*. Available at <http://www.gmc-uk.org/standards/secret.htm> (accessed 5 November 2003).

Genetic Interest Group (1999) *Genetic Testing, Screening and Eugenics'*, Genetic Interest Group Policy Paper. November. Available at <http://www.gig.org.uk/docs/gig_eugenics.pdf> (accessed 5 January 2004).

GeneWatch UK (2001) *Comments on the Report of the UK Population Biomedical Collection Protocol Development Workshop*, Buxton, UK: GeneWatch.

Gibson, L. and Cooke, R. (1959) 'A test for concentration of electrolytes in sweat in cystic fibrosis of the pancreas utilizing pilocarpine by iontophoresis', *Pediatrics*, 23: 545–9.

Giddens, A. (1990) *The Consequences of Modernity*, Cambridge: Polity Press.

Glasner, P. (2001) 'Rights or rituals? Why juries can do more harm than good', *PLA Notes*, 40: 43–5.

Golinski, J. (1998) *Making Natural Knowledge: Constructivism and the History of Science*, Cambridge: Cambridge University Press.

Gordon, J. (1999) 'Genetic advancement in humans', *Science*, 283: 2023–4.

Gottweis, H. (2002) 'The governance of genomics', *Critical Public Health*, 12:3, 207–20.

Greely, H. (1999) 'Breaking the stalemate: a prospective regulatory framework for unforeseen research uses of human tissue samples and health information', *Wake Forest Law Review*, 34: 737–66.

Green, J. (1995) 'Obstetricians' views on prenatal diagnosis and termination of pregnancy: 1980 compared with 1993', *British Journal of Obstetrics and Gynaecology*, 102: 228–32.

Green, S. (2003) ' "What do you mean 'what's wrong with her?' ": stigma and the lives of families of children with disabilities', *Social Science and Medicine*, 57:8, 1361–74.

Habermas, J. (2002) *The Future of Human Nature*, Cambridge: Polity Press.

Hall, S. (1996) 'Introduction: who needs identity?', in S. Hall and P. Du Gay (eds) *Questions of Cultural Identity*, London: Sage: 1–17.

Hallowell, N. (1999) 'Doing the right thing: genetic risk and responsibility', *Sociology of Health and Illness*, 21:5, 597–621.

—— and Richards, M. (1997) 'Understanding life's lottery: an evaluation of studies of genetic risk awareness', *Journal of Health Psychology*, 2:1, 31–43.

—— and Lawton, J. (2002) 'Negotiating present and future selves: managing the risk of hereditary ovarian cancer by prophylactic surgery', *Health*, 6:4, 423–43.

Harris, J. (1993) 'Is gene therapy a form of eugenics?', *Bioethics*, 7:2–3, 178–87.

Health and Social Care Act 2001, (c. 15) London: The Stationary Office Ltd, HMSO.

Hoeyer, K. (2002) 'Conflicting notions of personhood in genetic research', *Anthropology Today*, 18:5, 9–13.

—— (2004) 'Ambiguous gifts. Public anxiety, informed consent and commercial genetic biobank research', in R. Tutton and O. Corrigan (eds) *Genetic Databases: Socio-Ethical Issues in the Collection and Use of DNA*, London: Routledge, chapter 6, 97–116.

Holtzman, N. and Rothstein, M. (1992) 'Eugenics and genetic discrimination', invited editorial, *American Journal of Human Genetics*, 50: 457–9.

—— and Shapiro, D. (1998) 'Genetic testing and public policy', *British Medical Journal*, 316: 852–6.

House of Lords Select Committee on Science and Technology (2000) *Science and Society*, Third Report, Session 1999–2000. HL Paper 38, London: The Stationery Office. Available at <http://www.publications.parliament.uk/pa/ld199900/ldselect/ldsctech/38/3801.htm> (accessed 22 December 2003).

Hubbard, R. (1997) 'Abortion and disability: who should and who should not inhabit the world?', in L. Davis (ed.) *The Disability Studies Reader*, New York: Routledge.

Hubbard, R. and Newman, S. (2002) 'Yuppie eugenics: creating a world with genetic have and have-nots', *Z Magazine*, March. Available at <http://www.zmag.org/ZMag/articles/march02hubbard-newman.htm> (accessed 5 January 2004).

HUGO Ethics Committee (1998) *Statement on DNA Sampling: Control and Access*, London: Human Genome Organisation. Available at <http://www.gene.ucl.ac.uk/hugo/sampling.html> (accessed 5 November 2003).

Human Fertilisation and Embryology Authority (2003) *Sex Selection: Options for Regulation*. London: Human Fertilisation and Embryology Authority. Available at <http://www.hfea.gov.uk/AboutHFEA/Consultations/Final%20sex%20selection%20main%20report.pdf> (accessed 5 January 2004).

Human Genetics Commission (2002) *Inside Information: Balancing Interests in the Use of Personal Genetic Data*, London: Department of Health.

—— (2003) *Insurance, Genetics and Fairness – What Next After the Moratorium?*, Joint Meeting of Human Genetics Commission and Genetics and Insurance Committee, London, 22 September 2003. Available at <http://www.hgc.gov.uk/business_press23.htm> (accessed 22 December 2003).

Irwin, A. (2001) 'Constructing the scientific citizen: science and democracy in the biosciences', *Public Understanding of Science*, 10: 1–18.

—— and Michael, M. (2003) *Science, Social Theory and Public Knowledge*, Maidenhead: Open University Press; McGraw-Hill.

Jallinoja, P. (2001) 'Genetic screening in maternity care: preventive aims and voluntary choices', *Sociology of Health and Illness*, 23:3, 286–307.

Jasanoff, S. (1990) *The Fifth Branch: Science Advisors as Policymakers*, Cambridge, MA: Harvard University Press.

—— (2003) 'Breaking the waves in science studies: comment on H.M. Collins and Robert Evans, "The Third Wave of Science Studies" ', *Social Studies of Science*, 33:3, 389–400.

Johanson, R., Burr, R., Leighton, N. and Jones, P. (2000) 'Informed choice? Evidence of the persuasive power of professionals', *Journal of Public Health Medicine*, 22:3, 439–40.

Kaplan, J. (2000) *The Limits and Lies of Human Genetic Research Dangers for Social Policy*, New York: Routledge.

Kass, L. (2003) 'Ageless bodies, happy souls: biotechnology and the pursuit of perfection', *The New Atlantis*, 1: 1–11.

Kaye, H. (1997) *The Social Meaning of Modern Biology: From Social Darwinism to Sociobiology*, New Brunswick, NJ: Transaction.

Kaye, J. and Martin, P. (2000) 'Safeguards for research using large scale DNA collections', *British Medical Journal*, 321:7269, 1146–8.

Keller, E. (1985) *Reflections on Gender and Science*, New Haven: Yale University Press.

—— (2000) *The Century of the Gene*, Cambridge, MA: Harvard University Press.

Kelly, S. (2003) 'Public bioethics and publics: consensus, boundaries and participation in biomedical science policy', *Science, Technology & Human Values*, 28:3, 339–64.

Kenen, R., Ardern-Jones, A. and Eeles, R. (2003) 'Living with chronic risk: healthy women with a family history of breast/ovarian cancer', *Health Risk and Society*, 5:3, 315–32.

Kerr, A. (2000) '(Re)constructing genetic disease: the clinical continuum between cystic fibrosis and male infertility', *Social Studies of Science*, 30:6, 847–94.

—— (2003) 'Rights and responsibilities in the new genetics era', *Critical Social Policy*, 23:2, 208–26.

—— and Cunningham-Burley, S. (2000) 'On ambivalence and risk: reflexive modernity and the new human genetics', *Sociology*, 34:2, 283–304.

—— and Shakespeare, T. (2002) *Genetic Politics: From Eugenics to Genome*, Cheltenham: New Clarion Press.

—— Cunningham-Burley, S. and Amos, A. (1998a) 'Eugenics and the new genetics in Britain: examining contemporary professionals' accounts', *Science, Technology & Human Values*, 23:2, 175–98.

—— (1998b) 'Drawing the line: an analysis of lay people's discussions about the new human genetics', *Public Understanding of Science*, 7:2, 113–33.

—— (1998c) 'The new human genetics and health: mobilising lay expertise', *Public Understanding of Science*, 7:1, 41–60.

Kevles, D. (1995) *In the Name of Eugenics*, Cambridge, MA: Harvard University Press.

Kitzinger, J. and Williams, C. (2004) 'Colonising the future: legitimising hope and calming fears in the embryo stem cell debate', paper presented at 'First Lancaster-Cardiff CESAGen International Conference: Genomics and Society', London, 2–3 March.

Kleinman, D.L. (1998) 'Untangling Context: understanding a university laboratory in the commercial world', *Science, Technology & Human Values*, 23:3, 285–314.

Koch, L. and Stemerding, D. (1994) 'The sociology of entrenchment: a cystic fibrosis test for everyone?', *Social Science and Medicine*, 39:9, 1211–20.

Kulczycki, L. and MacLeod, K. (1961) 'Cystic fibrosis: a community challenge', *Public Health Reports*, 76: 85–90.

Lane, B., Williamson, P., Dodge, J.A., Harris, H., Super, M. and Harris, R. (1997) 'Confidential inquiry into families with two siblings with cystic fibrosis', *Archives of Diseases in Childhood*, 77, 501–3.

Lambert, H. and Rose, H. (1996) 'Disembodied knowledge? Making sense of medical knowledge', in A. Irwin and M. Michael (eds) *Misunderstanding Science: Making Sense of Science and Technology within Everyday Life*, Cambridge, MA: Cambridge University Press, 65–83.

Larson, E. (1998) 'Reframing the meaning of disability to families: the embrace of paradox', *Social Science and Medicine*, 47: 865–75.

Latour, B. (2000) 'When things strike back: a possible contribution of "science studies" to the social sciences', *British Journal of Sociology*, 1:5, 107–23.

—— (2003) 'Is re-modernization occuring – and if so, how to prove it? A commentary on Ulrich Beck', *Theory, Culture and Society*, 20:2, 35–48.

Lavery, S., Aurell, R., Turner, C., Castello, C., Veiga, A., Barri, P. and Winston, R. (2002) 'Preimplantation genetic diagnosis: patients' experiences and attitudes', *Human Reproduction*, 17:9, 2464–67.

Lawton, J. (2003) 'Lay experiences of health and illness: past research and future Agendas', *Sociology of Health and Illness*, 25:3, 23–40.

Lenaghan, J. (1999) *Brave New NHS? The Impact of the New Genetics on the Health Service*, London: IPPR.

Levitas, R. (1990) *The Concept of Utopia*, New York: Philip Allan.

Lewontin, R.C. (1991) *The Doctrine of DNA: Biology as Ideology*, London: Penguin.

Lippman, A. (1986) 'Access to prenatal screening: who decides?', *Canadian Journal of Women and the Law*, 1:2, 434–5.

—— (1991) 'Prenatal genetic testing and screening: constructing needs and reinforcing inequities', *American Journal of Law and Medicine*, 17: 15–50.

—— (1999a) 'Choice as a risk to women's health', *Health, Risk and Society*, 1:3, 281–92.

—— (1999b) 'Prenatal diagnosis', *American Journal of Public Health*, 89:10, 1592.

Lowe, C., May, C. and Reed, S. (1949) 'Fibrosis of pancreas in infants and children; a statistical study of clinician and hereditary features', *American Journal of Diseases of Children*, 78: 349–74.

Lowton, K. and Gabe, J. (2003) 'Life on a slippery slope: perceptions of health in adults with cystic fibrosis', *Sociology of Health and Illness*, 25:4, 281–319.

Lyttle, J. (1997) 'Is informed consent possible in the rapidly evolving world of DNA sampling?', *Canadian Medical Association Journal*, 156:2, 257–8.

McGee, G. (1997) *The Perfect Baby: A Pragmatic Approach to Genetics*, London: Rowman & Littlefield.

McGue, M. and Bouchard, T.J. Jr (1998) 'Genetic and environmental influences on human behavioral differences', *Annual Review of Neuroscience*, 21: 1–24.

McInnis, M. (1999) 'The assent of a nation: genethics and Iceland', *Clinical Genetics*, 55: 234–9.

McQueen, M. (1998) 'Ethical and legal issues in the procurement, storage and use of DNA', *Clinical Chemistry and Laboratory Medicine*, 36:8, 54–9.

Mann, C. (1994) 'Behavioural genetics in transition', *Science*, 264: 1686–9.

Marteau, T. and Richards, M. (1996) *The Troubled Helix: Social and Psychological Implications of the New Human Genetics*, Cambridge, MA: Cambridge University Press.

—— and Croyle, R. (1998) 'Psychological responses to genetic testing', *British Medical Journal*, 316:7132, 693–8.

—— and Dormandy, E. (2001) 'Facilitating informed choice in prenatal testing: how well are we doing?', *American Journal of Medical Genetics*, 106: 185–90.

——, Plenicar, M. and Kidd, J. (1993) 'Obstetricians presenting amniocentesis to pregnant women: practice observed', *Journal of Reproductive and Infant Psychology*, 11:1, 3–10.

Martin, P. (1999) 'Genes as drugs: the social shaping of gene therapy and the reconstruction of genetic disease', *Sociology of Health and Illness*, 21:5, 517–38.

Medical Research Council (2001) *Human Tissue and Biological Samples for use in Research: operational and ethical guidelines*, MRC Ethics Series, London: Medical Research Council.

Meek, J. (2002) 'Decode was meant to save lives . . . now it's destroying them', *The Guardian*, 31 October.

Merchant, C. (1980) *The Death of Nature: Women, Ecology, and the Scientific Revolution*, San Francisco: Harper and Row.

Merz, J. (1997) 'Psychosocial risks of storing and using human tissues in research', *Risk, Health, Safety and Environment*, 8: 235–48.

——, Magnus, D., Cho, M. and Caplan, A. (2002) 'Protecting subjects' interests in genetics research', *American Journal of Human Genetics*, 70: 965–71.

MORI (1999) *Public Support for Controversial Technologies Could Increase if Applications are Explained*. Available at <http://www.mori.com/polls/1999/novartis.shtml> (accessed 23 December 2003).

—— (2000) *Genetics Poll Shows Public's Confusion* 12th March 2000 Available at <http://www.mori.com/polls/2000/action.shtml> (accessed 12 January 2004).

Morris, J. (ed.) (1996) *Encounters with Strangers Feminism and Disability*, London: The Women's Press.

Mulderij, K. (1996) 'Research into the lifeworld of physically disabled children', *Child care, Health and Development*, 22:5, 311–22.

Mulkay, M. (1997) *The Embryo Research Debate: Science and the Politics of Reproduction*, Cambridge: Cambridge University Press.

Murray, J. and Cornell, C. (1981) 'Parentalplegia', *Psychology in Schools*, 18: 201–207.

National Screening Committee (2003) *Antenatal Screening for Down's Syndrome – National Guidance on Policy and Quality Management*. Available at <http://www.nelh.nhs.uk/screening/dssp/Guidancepolqual.pdf> (accessed 3 November 2003).

Nelkin, D. (2001) 'Anything for an edge: breeding a race of champions by germline', *Times Literary Supplement*, 19 October.

Nelkin, D. and Lindee, M. (1995) *The DNA Mystique: The Gene as a Cultural Icon*, New York: Freeman.

Nerlich, B. and Clarke, D. (2003) 'Anatomy of a media event: how arguments clashed in the 2001 human cloning debate', *New Genetics and Society*, 22:1, 43–60.

——, Clarke, D. and Dingwall, R. (1999) 'The influence of popular cultural imagery on public attitudes towards cloning', *Sociological Research Online*, 4:3. Available at <http://www.socresonline.org.uk/4/3/nerlich.html> (accessed 18 December 2003).

Nerlich, B., Dingwall, R. and Clarke, D. (2002) 'The book of life: how the completion of the Human Genome Project was revealed to the public', *Health*, 6:4, 445–69.

Novas, C. and Rose, N. (2000) 'Genetic risk and the birth of the somatic individual', *Economy and Society*, special issue on Configurations of Risk, 29:4, 484–513.

Office of Science and Technology (2000) *Excellence and Opportunity: A Science and Innovation Policy for the 21st Century*, Stationery Office Ltd. Available at <http://www.ost.gov.uk/enterprise/dtiwhite/index.html> (accessed 22 December 2003).

Office of Science and Technology and The Wellcome Trust (2000) *Science and the Public: A Review of Science Communication and Public Attitudes to Science in Britain*. Available at <http://www.wellcome.ac.uk/en/images/sciencepublic_3391.pdf> (accessed 22 December 2003).

Pálsson, G. and Harðardóttir, K. (2002) 'For whom the cell tolls: debates about Biomedicine', *Current Anthropology*, 43:2, 271–301.

Parens, E. and Asch, A. (eds) (2000) *Prenatal Testing and Disability Rights*, Hastings Center Studies in Ethics, series edited by M. Hanson and D. Callaman, Washington, DC: Georgetown University Press.

Parsons, E. and Atkinson, P. (1992) 'Lay constructions of genetic risk', *Sociology of Health and Illness*, 14: 439–55.

Paul, D. (1992) 'Eugenic anxieties, social realities and political choices', *Social Research*, 59:3, 663–83.

—— (1998) *Controlling Human Heredity: 1865 to the Present*, Amhurst, NY: Humanity Press.

Pelchart, D., Lefebvre, H. and Perreault, M. (2003) 'Differences and similarities between mothers' and fathers' experiences of caring for a child with a disability', *Journal of Child Health Care*, 7:4, 231–47.

People Science and Policy Ltd. (2002) *BioBank UK: A Question of Trust: A Consultation Exploring and Addressing Questions of Public Trust*, London: Medical Research Council; Wellcome Trust.

Petersen, A. (1999) 'Counselling the genetically "at-risk": a critique of "non-directiveness"', *Health Risk and Society*, 1:3, 253–66.

—— (2002) 'Replicating our bodies, losing our selves: news media portrayals of human cloning in the wake of Dolly', *Body & Society*, 8:4, 71–90.

—— and Bunton, R. (2002) *The New Genetics and the Public's Health*, London: Routledge.

Rabeharisoa, V. and Callon, M. (2002) 'The involvement of patients' associations in research', *International Social Science Journal*, 54:1, 57–67.

Rabinow, P. (1996) *Essays on the Anthropology of Reason*, Chichester, NJ: Princeton University Press.

—— (1999) *French DNA: trouble in purgatory*, Chicago, IL: University of Chicago Press.

Rapp, R. (1994) 'Women's responses to prenatal diagnosis: a sociocultural perspective on diversity', in K. Rothenberg and E. Thomson (eds) *Women and Prenatal Testing: facing the challenges of technology*, Columbus, OH: Ohio State University Press, 219–33.

—— (2000) *Testing Women, Testing the Fetus, the social impact of amniocentesis in America*, New York: Routledge.

Reilly, P. and Page, D. (1998) 'We're off to see the genome', *Nature Genetics*, 20, Sept., 15–17.

Reindal, S. (2000) 'Disability, gene therapy and eugenics – a challenge to John Harris', *Journal of Medical Ethics*, 26: 89–94.

Resnik, D. and Langer, P. (2001) 'Human germline gene therapy reconsidered', *Human Gene Therapy*, 12:11, 1449–58.

Reynolds, T. (2003) 'Down's Syndrome screening is unethical: views of today's research ethics committees', *Journal of Clinical Pathology*, 56: 268–70.

Rifkin, J. (2001) 'Will companies hold control of life made in a petri dish?', *Los Angeles Times*, 23 July. Available at <http://www.commondreams.org/> (accessed 5 January 2004).

Rimmer, M. (2003) 'Myriad genetics: patent law and genetic testing', *European Intellectual Property Law*, 25:1, 20–33.

Roberts, L. (1988a) 'The race for the cystic fibrosis gene', *Science*, 240: 141–4.

—— (1988b) 'The race for the cystic fibrosis gene nears end', *Science*, 240: 282–5.

Rock, P. (1996) 'Eugenics and euthanasia: a cause for concern for disabled people, particularly disabled women', *Disability and Society*, 11:1, 121–8.

Rommens, J., Iannuzzi, M., Kerem, B., Drumm, M., Melmer, G., Dean, M., Rozmahel, R., Cole, J., Kennedy, D., Hidaka, N., *et al.* (1989) 'Identification of the cystic fibrosis gene: chromosome walking and jumping', *Science*, 245: 1059–65.

Rose, N. (2000) 'The biology of culpability: pathological identity and crime control in a biological culture', *Theoretical Criminology*, 4:1, 5–34.

—— (2001) 'The politics of life itself', *Theory, Culture and Society*, 18:6, 1–30.

Rothman, B. (1988) *The Tentative Pregnancy: Amniocentesis and the Sexual Politics of Motherhood*, London: Pandora.

—— (1998) *Genetic Maps and Human Imaginations: The Limits of Science in Understanding Who We Are*, New York: W. W. Norton and Co. Inc.

Rothstein, M. (2002) 'The role of IRB's in research involving commercial biobanks', *Journal of Law, Medicine and Ethics*, 30: 105–8.

Royal Society, The (2003) *Royal Society National Forum for Science 2003 (People's Science Summit): Genetic Testing – Which Way Forward?*, London: The Royal Society. Available at <http://www.royalsoc.ac.uk/scienceinsociety/data/forum/ForumGeneticTest2003.pdf> (accessed 18 December 2003).

Savulescu, J. (2001) 'Is current practice around late termination of pregnancy eugenic and discriminatory? Maternal interests and abortion', *Journal of Medical Ethics*, 27: 165–71.

—— (2002) 'Deaf lesbians, "designer disability" and the future of medicine', *British Medical Journal*, 325: 771–3.

Shakespeare, T. (1995) 'Back to the future? New genetics and disabled people', *Critical Social Policy*, 44:5, 22–35.

—— (1999) ' "Losing the plot?" Medical and activist discourses of contemporary genetics and disability', *Sociology of Health and Illness*, 21:5, 669–88.

——, Gillespie-Sells, K. and Davies, D. (1996) *The Sexual Politics of Disability: Untold Desires*, London: Cassell.

Sharp, K. and Earle, S. (2002) 'Feminism, abortion and disability: irreconcilable differences?', *Disability and Society*, 7:2, 137–46.

Sharp, R. and Foster, M. (2002) 'Community involvement in the ethical review of genetic research: lessons from American Indian and Alaska native populations', *Environmental Health Perspectives*, 110: suppl. 2, 145–8.

Shepherd, M., Hattersley, A. and Sparkes, A. (2000) 'Predictive genetic testing in diabetes: a case study of multiple perspectives', *Qualitative Health Research*, 10:2, 242–59.

Shiloh, S. (1996) 'Decision-making in the context of genetic risk', in T. Marteau and M. Richards (eds) *The Troubled Helix: Social and Psychological Implications of the New Human Genetics*, Cambridge: Cambridge University Press, 82–103.

Silver, L. (1997) *Remaking Eden: Cloning and Beyond in a Brave New World*, New York: Avon Books.

Smaglik, P. (2000) 'Tissue donors use their influence in deal over gene patent terms', *Nature*, 407:6806, 821.

Smith, C. (2002) 'The sequestration of experience: rights talk and moral thinking in "late modernity" ', *Sociology*, 36:1, 43–66.

Spencer, K., Coombes, E., Mallard, A. and Milford-Ward, A. (1992) 'Free beta human choriogonadotropin in Down's syndrome screening: a multicentre study of its role compared with other biochemical markers', *Annals of Clinical Biochemistry*, 29: 506–18.

——, Spencer, C., Power, M., Dawson, C. and Nicolaides, K. (2003) 'Screening for chromosomal abnormalities in the first trimester using ultrasound and maternal serum biochemistry in a one-stop clinic: a review of three years prospective experience', *British Journal of Obstetrics and Gynaecology*, 110: 281–6.

Staley, K. (2001) *Giving Your Genes to Biobank UK: Questions to Ask*. Report for GeneWatch UK, Buxton: GeneWatch UK.

Staples, S. (2000) 'Human Resource: Newfoundland's 300-year-old genetic legacy has triggered a gold rush', *Business Magazine*, 17:3, 117–20.

Stegmayr, B. and Asplund, K. (2002) 'Informed consent for genetic research on blood stored for more than a decade: a population based study', *British Medical Journal*, 325:21, 634–5.

Stewart, J., Kendall, E. and Coote, A. (1995) *A Citizens' Juries*, London: Institute of Public Policy Research.

Stiker, H.-J. (1999) *Corps Infirmes et Sociétés*; trans. William Sayers (1999) *A History of Disability*, Ann Arbour, MI: University of Michigan Press.

Stock, G. (2002) *Redesigning Humans: Our Inevitable Genetic Future*, New York: Houghton Mifflin.

Stockdale, A. (1999) 'Waiting for the cure: mapping the social relations of human gene therapy research', *Sociology of Health and Illness*, 21:5, 579–96.

Sulston, J. and Ferry, G. (2002) *The Common Thread: A Story of Science, Politics, Ethics and the Human Genome*, London: Bantam Press.

Super, M. (1992) 'Milestones in cystic fibrosis', *British Medical Bulletin*, 48:4, 717–37.

Taanila, L., Syrjälä, J., Kokkonen, J. and Järvelin, M-R. (2002) 'Coping of parents with physically and/or intellectually disabled children', *Child Care, Health and Development* 28:1, 73–86.

Tanner, J. (2002) 'Parental separation and divorce: can we provide an ounce of prevention?', *Pediatrics*, November.

Tauber, A. and Sarkar, S. (1992) 'The Human Genome Project: has blind reductionism gone too far', *Perspectives in Biology and Medicine*, 35:2, 220–35.

Thomas, C. (1999) *Female Forms Experiencing and Understanding Disability*, Oxford: Oxford University Press.

Thompson, R., Gil, K., Gustafson, K., George, L., Keith, B., Spock, A. and Kinney, T. (1994) 'Stability and change in the psychological adjustment of mothers of children and adolescents with cystic fibrosis and sickle cell disease', *Journal of Pediatric Psychology*, 19: 171–88.

——, Hodges, K. and Hamlett, K. (1990) 'A matched comparison of adjustment in children with Cystic Fibrosis and psychiatrically referred and nonreferred children', *Journal of Pediatric Psychology*, 15: 745–9.

Thomson, M. (1998) *The Problem of Mental Deficiency: Eugenics, Democracy and Social Policy in Britain c. 1870–1959*, Oxford: Clarendon Press.

Trombley, S. (1988) *The Right to Reproduce: A History of Coercive Sterilization*, London: Weidenfeld and Nicolson.

Turner, G. and Wynne, B. (1992) 'Risk communication', in J. Durant (ed.) *Biotechnology in Public: A Review of Recent Research*, London: Science Museum, 109–41.

UK Stem Cell Bank Steering Committee. Available at <http://www.mrc. ac.uk/index/strategy-strategy/strategy-science_strategy/strategy-strategy_ implementation/strategy-government_spending_review_initiatives/strategy- stem_cells/strategy-stem_cell_governance/public-stemcell_governance_ steering.htm#anch-public-stemcell_governance_steering-Anchor1> (accessed 22 December 2003).

Van Dijck, J. (1998) *Imagenation: Popular Images of Genetics*, London: Macmillan.

Verity, C. and Nicoll, A. (2002) 'Consent, Confidentiality and the Threat to Public Health Surveillance', *British Medical Journal*, 324: 1210–13.

Ville, I., Ravaauld, J., Diard, C. and Paicheler, H. (1994) 'Self-representations and physical impairment: a social constructivist approach', *Sociology of Health and Illness*, 16: 301–21.

Wald, N., Hackshaw, A., Haddow, J., Palomaki, G. and Knight, G. (1993) 'Use of free β-hCG in Down's syndrome screening', *Annals of Clinical Biochemistry*, 30: 512–18.

——, Kennard, A., Hackshaw, A. and McGuire, A. (1998) 'Antenatal screening for Down's Syndrome', *Health Technology Assessment Report*, 2:1.

——, Rodeck, C., Hackshaw, A., Walters, J., Chitty, L. and Mackinson, A. (2003) 'First and second trimester antenatal screening for Down's syndrome: the results of the Serum, Urine and Ultrasound Screening Study (SURUSS)', *Health Technology Assessment*, 7:11, 51 pages.

Waldby, C. (2002) 'Stem cells, tissue cultures and the production of biovalue', *Health*, 6:3, 305–24.

Walsh, V. (2002) 'Biotechnology and the UK 2000–05: globalization and innovation', *New Genetics and Society*, 21:2, 149–76.

Warner, M. (2002) *Publics and Counterpublics*, New York: Zone Books.

Webster, A. (2002) 'Innovative Health Technologies and the social: redefining health, medicine and the body', *Current Sociology*, 50:3, 443–57.

—— and Nelis, A. (1999) 'Regulating the gene: from genetic consumption to regulatory trust', *Health, Risk and Society*, 1:3, 301–12.

Wellcome Trust, The (1998) *Public Perspectives on Human Cloning: A Social Research Study*, London: The Wellcome Trust. Available at <http://www.wellcome.ac.uk/ en/images/cloning_report_slimversion_2816.pdf> (accessed 23 December 2003).

Welsh Institute for Health and Social Care (1998) *What Conditions Should Be Fulfilled Before Genetic Testing for Susceptibility to Common Diseases Becomes Widely Available on the NHS?*, Pontypridd: University of Glamorgan. Available at <http://www.phgu.org.uk/info_database/testing_etc/summary%20rec> (accessed 22 December 2003).

Welshman, J. (1996) 'In search of the "problem family": public health and social work in England and Wales 1940–70', *Social History of Medicine*, 9:3, 447–65.

Whittle, M. (2001) 'Down's Syndrome screening: where to now?', *British Journal of Obstetrics and Gynaecology*, 108: 544–61.

WHO (1998) 'Proposed International Guidelines on Ethical Issues in Medical Genetics and Genetic Services'. Report of a WHO Metting on Ethical Issues in Medical Genetics, Geneva, 15–16 December 1997, World Health Organization, Geneva.

Wieting, S. (2002) 'Public and private priorities in managing time in genetic research: the Icelandic deCode case', *Symbolic Interaction*, 25:3, 271–87.

Wilkie, T. (1993) *Perilous knowledge*, London: Farbes and Farber.

Williams, C., Alderson, P. and Farsides, B. (2002a) ' "Drawing the line" in prenatal screening and testing: health practitioners' discussions', *Health, Risk and Society*, 4: 61–75.

—— (2002b) 'Too many choices? Hospital and community staff reflect on the future of prenatal screening', *Social Science and Medicine*, 55: 743–53.

Williams, C., Kitzinger, J. and Henderson, L. (2003) 'Envisaging the embryo in stem cell research: rhetorical strategies and media reporting of the ethical debates', *Sociology of Health and Illness*, 25:7, 793–814.

Williams, G. (1984) 'The genesis of chronic illness: narrative reconstruction', *Sociology of Health and Illness*, 6:2, 175–200.

Winston, R. and Hardy, K. (2002) 'Are we ignoring potential dangers of *in vitro* fertilization and related treatment?', *Nature Cell Biology and Nature Medicine Fertility Supplement*, s14–18.

Woolgar, S. and Cooper, G. (1999) 'Do artefacts have ambivalence? Moses' bridges, winner's bridges and other urban legends in S and TS', *Social Studies of Science*, 29:3, 433–49.

World Medical Association (2002) *Declaration on Ethical Considerations Regarding Health Databases*. Available at <http://www.wma.net/e/policy/d1.htm> (accessed 10 November 2003).

Wright, S. (1986) 'Recombinant DNA technology and its social transformation, 1972–1982, *OSIRIS*, 2nd series, 2: 303–60.

Wynne, B. (1995) 'The public understanding of science', in S. Jasanoff, G. Markel, J. Petersen and T. Pinch (eds), *Handbook of Science and Technology Studies*, London: Sage, 361–88.

—— (2003) 'Seasick on the Third Wave? Subverting the hegemony of propositionalism: response to Collins & Evans (2002)', *Social Studies of Science*, 33:3, 401–17.

Index

abortion 21, 23, 24, 57, 64, 67, 71, 72, 81,
  83, 158; legislation 17, 64
accountability 7, 168
Action Research 129
Ahmad, W. 84
Albert, B. 69–70
alcoholism 39
Alderson, P. 5, 66, 72, 74, 79
Allen, G. 18
alpha fetoprotein screening 64
altruism 107, 115, 116
Alzheimer's disease 52, 130
Alzheimer's Society, Quality Research in
  Dementia (QRD) Advisory Network
  52–3
amniocentesis 22, 64, 65, 77, 133
Andersen, D. 58
Anderson, R. 114
Anderton, J. 98
Anionwu, E. 84
anonymity of data 112, 114
antenatal screening see prenatal,
  screening
antenatal testing see prenatal, testing
anti-abortion movement 31
Antonellis, A. 41
Ardern-Jones, A. 91
Asch, A. 84, 99, 101
Ashcroft, R. 144, 152–3
Asplund, K. 120
assisted conception 2, 32, 57, 65
Association Français contre les Myopathies
  (AFM) 51
Atkin, K. 84, 99, 101
Atkinson, P. 62, 81, 92, 132
autonomy 16, 19, 22, 32, 57, 71, 73,
  152, 169
Avon Longitudinal Study of Parents and
  Children (ALSPAC) 104, 120, 139

Bailey, R. 17
Balmer, B. 48–9
Barbero, G. 59
Barbour, V. 105, 114
Batchelor, C. 54, 62, 168
Bauman, Z. 72
BCODP, International Sub-Committee 35
Beaudry, P. 59
Beck, U. 5, 30, 134–5
behavioural genetics 21, 33, 34, 36, 53
beneficence 32, 73
Berg, K. 108, 114
Beskow, L. 106
Billings, P. 33
Bindra, R. 75
Binet test 19
biobanks 3, 7, 12, 13, 33, 103–23, 148,
  156, 166; research 10, 13, 110, 115,
  119, 148, 166
bioethics 73, 74, 106, 148, 149, 150, 152,
  154, 157, 163; public 148–54, 157
biofutures 148, 149–50, 152–3
biography narratives 89–94
BioIndustry Association 147
biomedicine 17, 73, 95, 106, 110, 120,
  125, 147, 152, 154–6, 159
biopiracy 117
biopolitics 144
Black, E. 35
black boxing 47–8, 49, 62, 137, 163, 166
Bobrow, M. 29
Bodmer, W. 28
Bonnefort, J. 60
Bouchard, T.J. Jr 22
Bourdieu, P. 126, 128
Braude, P. 66
breast cancer 2, 39, 68, 85, 91, 94, 96, 99,
  100, 114
British Mental Health Act (1959) 21

Brock, D. 17
Brown, N. 144
Brunger, F. 80
Bunton, R. 135
Bury, M. 8, 85, 94
Busby, H. 107

Callon, M. 52, 135
Cambrosio, A. 146
campaigning organizations 2, 94, 98, 106, 110, 118, 147, 164
cancer 2, 8, 33, 84, 91, 94, 95, 99, 103, 104, 112, 113
capitalism 22, 31, 43, 118, 151, 163
Caplan, A. 70, 150
Catholic Church 20
Caulfield, T. 108
Caygill, H. 144
Celera 44, 46, 49
cell lines 11, 50, 51, 117, 139, 159
Center for Bioethics, University of Pennsylvania 150
Centre d'Etude du Polymorphisme Humain (CEPH) 51
CF History Project 58–60, 67–8
Chakravarti, A. 24
Chapman, E. 84
Chapple, J. 23–4
Charcot-Marie-Tooth disease (CMT) 40–3, 49, 50, 56, 62
Charmaz, K. 8, 85
Chief Medical Officer's Expert Group 159
choice 1, 2, 3, 4, 5, 6, 12, 13, 16, 17, 18, 20, 22, 23, 24, 27, 29, 31, 32, 35, 36, 64, 66, 67, 68, 69, 70, 71, 72, 73, 74, 75, 76, 79, 82, 83, 91, 94, 97, 108, 112, 131, 146, 151, 152, 153, 159, 162, 163, 166, 169; individual 1, 5, 6, 10, 15, 24, 30, 33, 36, 64, 66, 67, 68, 69, 70, 71, 72, 73, 74, 82, 103, 106, 117, 153, 156, 162, 163, 169; informed 6, 30, 68, 69, 70, 75, 79
chorionic villus sampling 65
Christian Medical Fellowship 70
chromosomal abnormalities 23, 64, 65, 76
Chrysanthou, M. 144
citizen-consumers 128, 131
citizens' juries 136, 137–8
citizenship 12, 21, 30, 53, 71, 157, 159; active 110, 124, 134–8
Clarke, A. 6, 72, 83
clinical genetics 2, 33
clinical practice 2, 8, 10, 11, 14, 15, 43, 52, 110, 113, 116, 133, 145, 167, 168
clinical services 6

cloning 31, 143, 144, 149, 156, 157–8, 159, 160, 163
coercion 2, 16, 17, 18–22, 24, 27, 36, 70, 71, 74, 82, 143
cognitive ability 21
collaboration (between professionals) 14, 29, 40, 52, 53, 54, 55, 56, 62, 85
Collaborative Research Inc. 55
Collins, F. 44
Collins, H. 140, 141
commerce 28–30, 162
commercial eugenics *see* eugenics, commercial
commercialization 46–9, 116–21
community involvement in research 119
competition (between professionals) 46, 49, 53–4, 56, 133
confidentiality 13, 30, 103, 104, 105, 107, 110, 111, 112, 113, 114, 115, 116, 120, 131
Conrad, P. 38–9, 158
consensus conferences 136, 138
consent: blanket 108; community 104, 109, 111; informed 13, 21, 76, 103, 104, 105, 108, 106–11, 112, 121, 155; presumed 104, 106
constructing citizens and publics 138–42
consumer choice 5, 29, 31, 36, 108, 153
Consumer Council, The 136
consumers 163
Cooke, R. 58
Cooper, G. 161
coping with risk 84, 92
Cornell, C. 87
cost benefit arguments 24, 76, 156
Cox, S. 84, 92, 98
Coyne, I. 87
Crick, F. 21
criminality 25
Croyle, R. 79
Cunningham-Burley, S. 5, 10, 17, 33, 34, 67, 71
cure 6, 52, 107, 110, 143, 146, 147, 148, 149, 154, 158, 159, 160, 162, 164, 166
Cyranoski, D. 117
cystic fibrosis (CF) 27, 55–6, 57–8, 65, 67–8, 73, 81, 84, 87, 88, 92–3, 133; gene 61, 62, 103; history of 12, 23, 58–60, 174
Cystic Fibrosis Trust 52

Data Protection Act (1998) 112
Davies, K. 55
Davies, P. 55

Davis 59
Davison, A. 125, 126, 129, 131
Dawson, C. 115
De Vries 25
deCode Genetics 104, 116, 118, 120
deficit model (public understanding of science) 124, 128, 132, 134, 142
degeneracy 19, 21, 22
dementia 52–3
democracy 5, 30, 32, 121, 132
Department of Health 33, 145, 148
Department of Trade and Industry 135
designer babies 144, 158
deviancy 15, 22, 162
diabetes 90, 120, 145
disability 16, 17, 21, 22, 23–4, 27, 32, 57, 70, 71, 72, 73, 81, 82, 83, 91, 98, 99, 137, 147; activists 139, 164; movement, activists 9, 17, 35, 53, 69, 91, 98, 139, 164; rights 2, 9, 69, 99; studies 9, 84
disabled people 9, 17, 18, 19, 22, 33, 35, 36, 51, 71, 72, 80, 81, 88, 101, 163
disclosure 111, 113
discovery 4, 10, 12, 21, 38–45, 47–8, 49, 50, 51, 53, 54, 55, 56, 61, 62, 64, 104, 163, 165
discrimination 33, 35, 36, 79, 85, 88, 105, 131, 162; genetic 100, 109, 110–11, 118, 151
disease: cause of 54; definitions of 56–62
distal spinal muscular atrophy (dSMA) 40–3, 49, 50, 56, 62
DNA 2, 13, 21, 24, 26, 29, 33, 39, 47, 51, 61, 65, 104, 105, 107, 112, 114, 117
Dodge, J. 23, 93
Donaldson report 159
donation 13, 52, 103, 104, 107, 120
Donis-Keller, H. 55
Dormandy, E. 6, 84
Down's syndrome 66, 83; screening in the UK 24, 64, 74–82
Duchenne muscular dystrophy 81
Dunkerley, D. 135
Durant, J. 128, 134

Earle, S. 71
Economic and Social Research Council (ESRC) 3
Eeles, R. 91
Einsiedel, E. 137
Eliasoph, N. 131, 138
embryo research 2, 30–1
emergent technologies 3, 10, 143
Engelhardt 32

enlightenment 4, 39, 43, 56, 58, 143, 144, 155, 162, 165
essentialism 55; *see also* genetic determinism; geneticization; reductionism
ethical capitalism 118–19
ethical review 50, 116, 121, 139
ethics 3, 5, 50–1, 62, 73, 106, 107, 109, 111, 112, 114, 116, 117, 120, 121, 148, 149, 150, 152, 154, 156, 165, 168
ethnic minorities 79, 101, 111, 137
eugenics 2, 4, 10, 15, 16, 19, 22, 25, 27, 67, 71, 73, 82, 106, 143, 154, 162; commercial 31; contemporary debates 4, 18, 30–6; *laissez-faire* 30, 32; movement 18; negative 19, 22
European Convention on Human Rights and Biomedicine 111, 115
euthanasia 17, 19, 20, 71, 149
Evans, G. 134
Evans, R. 140
Ewbank, J. 33
expert relations 53–6
expertise 28–30, 140, 164, 169
experts 10, 15, 20, 34, 35, 36, 37, 98, 109, 121, 123, 124–5, 131, 136, 137, 138, 139, 140, 141, 142, 146, 152, 164, 169

families 2, 8, 11, 16, 21, 22, 24, 25, 43, 54, 58, 59, 65, 67, 80, 81, 82, 84, 85, 86, 87, 88, 89, 90, 91, 92, 94, 95, 96, 97, 98, 99, 100, 101, 104, 105, 111, 112, 113, 121, 132, 133, 137
Fanconi, G. 58
Fanconi anaemia 65
Farsides, B. 5, 66, 72, 74, 79
fascism 17
fear 23, 33, 96, 97, 111, 123, 128, 136, 144, 151, 152, 156, 157, 158
Fears, R. 116
feedback to research participants 115
feminism 18
Ferguson, M. 86–7
Ferry, G. 29
Finkler, K. 84, 85, 95–7
Fleischer, M. 135–6
focus groups 115, 125, 134, 136, 138
Foster, M. 111, 119
Franklin, S. 50–1, 84, 156, 157, 168
Fujimura, J. 47, 54, 168
Fukuyama, F. 152, 154
funding agencies 3, 4, 11, 45, 49, 50, 52, 56, 62, 73, 145, 154, 162, 167

future(s) 1, 4, 5, 6, 9, 10, 11, 13, 16, 31, 33, 35, 43, 47, 81, 86, 92, 94, 98, 106, 108, 109, 111, 114, 136, 143–6, 148, 149, 150, 151, 152, 153, 154, 156, 157, 159, 160, 162–3

Gabe, J. 84, 88, 92
Galileo Genomics Inc 117
Galton 19
Garrod, A. 58
GARS gene 40–2, 44, 56, 62
gay gene 33, 158
General Medical Council 105, 112, 113
genes 1, 2, 5, 7, 8, 9, 10, 11, 12, 21, 22, 25, 27, 29, 35, 38, 39, 40, 41, 42, 43, 44, 48, 49, 53, 56, 58, 61, 62, 65, 95, 103, 104, 115, 145, 156, 157, 162, 163, 164, 165, 166, 167; chips 143; mapping 49; patenting 46, 47, 114, 120, 150; pool 16, 154–5; sequencing 46; therapy 33, 57, 62, 143, 145, 148, 156
genetic complexity 27, 166
genetic counselling 5, 23, 68, 71, 80, 83, 90, 94, 115
genetic databanks *see* biobanks
genetic determinism 7, 27, 30, 38, 151, 166
genetic diagnosis 36, 98; *see also* preimplantation genetic diagnosis
genetic disease 8, 9, 10, 55, 57, 62, 64, 84, 85, 86, 90, 92, 94, 96, 97, 99, 100, 101, 103, 115, 161, 166, 168
genetic enhancement 10, 31, 33, 143, 144, 151, 154, 155, 156, 160
genetic essentialism 25
genetic fitness 15
Genetic Interest Group (GIG) 34
genetic profiling 143, 147
genetic reductionism 24–8, 166
genetic research 3, 10, 11, 12, 13, 21, 30, 38, 39, 44, 46, 50, 53, 55, 98, 103, 104, 106, 107, 109, 116, 117, 120, 129, 147, 148, 166
genetic risk 35, 81, 90, 94, 95, 96, 97, 98, 100, 101, 102, 164
genetic screening 2, 10, 12, 24, 65, 66, 67, 70, 72, 75, 80, 82, 83, 99, 166; women's experiences of 11, 83
genetic services 10, 30, 33, 146
genetic solidarity 113
genetic technologies 1, 4, 5, 6, 12–13, 15, 16, 27, 32, 35, 37, 64, 101, 103, 124, 131, 132, 143, 144, 145, 151, 152, 156,

158, 161, 163, 167, 169; *see also* reproductive genetics
genetic testing 24, 62, 66, 68, 69, 80, 81, 83, 96, 97, 98, 100, 111, 133, 137, 147; attitudes towards 132
genetic tests 2, 66, 90, 151
genetic underclass 144
genetically modified organisms (GMOs) 129, 136
geneticists 4, 8, 16, 17, 20, 21, 24, 27, 28, 36, 38, 46, 60, 62, 64, 65, 67, 71, 99, 133
geneticization 24
genetics: contemporary 6, 10, 11, 15, 17, 18, 30, 164; medical 21, 34, 95, 97
GeneWatch UK 104, 110
genome mapping 49
genomics 50
genotype 27, 60
germline: gene therapy 154; genetic engineering 32
Geron Bio-Med 50–1
Gibson, L. 58
Giddens, A. 5
Glasner, P. 135, 137–8
GlaxoSmithCline 3
God 149, 150, 152
Golinski, J. 45
Gordon, J. 30, 155
Gottweis, H. 50
governance 13, 28–30, 50–3, 73, 103, 105, 106, 109, 116–21, 125, 136, 139, 150, 151, 152, 157, 162, 166, 167, 168, 169
government(s) 1, 2, 3, 5, 19, 28, 50, 53, 55, 67, 69, 104, 105, 110–11, 115, 118, 120, 125, 126, 128, 133, 134, 135, 136, 142, 143, 145, 146, 147, 148, 157
Greely, H. 108
Green, J. 6, 72
Green, S. 89

haemachromatosis 115
Hallowell, N. 84, 85–6, 94, 95
Harðardóttir, K. 120
Hardy, K. 65
Harris, J. 32
Health Care Trust 139
health consumers 12, 103
health service research 6
Health Technology Assessment programme 77
heart disease 2, 8, 104, 145
Hoeyer, K. 107, 108
Holtzman, N. 35, 79

Hood, L. 151
Hooper, J. 117
hope 66, 89, 93, 99, 107, 125, 151, 155, 156, 159
House of Lords Select Committee on Science and Technology 135
Hubbard, R. 5, 31, 70
Human Fertilization and Embryology Authority (HFEA) 32
Human Genetics Commission (HGC) 110–11, 113, 146, 147, 148, 169
Human Genetics Commission Consultative Panel 136
Human Genome Diversity Project 117
Human Genome Mapping Project (HGMP) 49, 120
Human Genome Organization (HUGO) 112
Human Genome Project (HGP) 2, 17, 25, 26, 27, 28, 46, 48–9, 50, 53, 166
Human Germ Line Genetic Manipulation (HGLM) 155
human nature 153, 157
Huntington's disease (HD) 84, 85, 97, 99–100, 111
Hussein, S. 157
hype 24, 151, 160, 163, 166

Icelandic government 104, 118, 120
Icelandic Health Sector Database 104, 106, 116, 117
Icelandic Medical Association 104
identity 11, 12, 25, 28, 51, 82, 90, 98, 111, 118, 139, 144, 147, 157, 158, 160, 162, 164–6
ignorance 12, 124, 152
immigration 18
impairment(s) 57, 87, 88, 89, 96, 101–2, 139, 158
in vitro fertilization (IVF) 2, 31, 51, 73
Indigenous Peoples Coalition on Biocolonialism 118
individualism 4, 21, 25, 36, 121
infertility 57, 60
informed consent *see* consent
informed debate 135
innovation(s) 4, 29, 45, 46, 47, 48, 136, 153
Innovative Health Technologies Programme 3
Institute of Public Policy Research (IPPR) 136
institutional reflexivity 7, 30, 82
instrumentation 61, 162
insurance 33, 35, 52, 69, 109, 110–11; companies 34–5, 110, 111

Integrated Test, the 75, 77
Intema Ltd 77
interpretive flexibility 114
interviews: in-depth 134
IQ 19
Irwin, A. 124, 125, 126, 128, 133, 135

Jallinoja, P. 66, 72
Jasanoff, S. 140, 168
Johanson, R. 6
Joseph, K. 21

Kaplan, J. 57
Kass, L. 149–50, 152, 153
Kaye, H. 25–6
Keller, E. 27, 39
Kelly, S. 148, 168, 169
Kenen, R. 91
Kennard, A. 24, 74
Kent, D. 101
Kerr, A. 5, 10, 33, 34, 60, 67, 71, 105, 106, 131, 133, 140
Kevles, D. 20, 23
King, Sir David 147
Kitzinger, J. 158, 159
Kleinman, D. 45, 48
Koch, L. 66, 73, 75, 82
Kulczycki, L. 59

laboratory practice(s) 3, 47–8, 168
Lambert, H. 92, 132–3
Landsteiner, K. 58
Lane, B. 81
Langer, P. 154–5
Larson, E. 88, 89
Latour, B. 7, 8, 168
Lavery, S. 65, 84
Lawton, J. 84, 85–6, 94, 95, 98, 99
lay expertise 137, 139–40
lay knowledge 132–4, 138
lay–expert divide 136, 137, 140, 168
Lenaghan, J. 136
Levitas, R. 144
liberty 37, 143, 159
Lindee, M. 19, 25
Lippman, A. 5, 72, 76, 79, 80
Little, P. 24
Local Research Ethics Committees (LRECs) 112, 116
Lowe, C. 58
Lowton, K. 84, 88, 92
Lyttle, J. 108

McGee, G. 150–2, 155
McGue, M. 22
McInnis, M. 106, 120
McKellin, W. 84, 92, 98
MacLeod, K. 59
McQueen, M. 108, 120
Mann, C. 21–2
Markens, S. 158
marketing 44, 53, 54, 62
Marteau, T. 6, 79, 84, 99, 100
Martin, P. 57
mass media 156–60, 163
maternity care 75
Mattaei 26
media 38–9, 49, 50, 55, 117, 120, 124,
    129, 140, 145, 152, 156, 157
Medical Research Council (MRC) 3
medicalization 21, 57, 95, 97, 157
Meek, J. 104
Melmer, G.
Mendel 25
Mendelianism 33
mental health 22
Merchant, C. 39
Merz, J. 107, 112, 116, 118, 119
Michael, M. 124, 125, 126, 133, 135
Milford-Ward, A.
Millennium Pharmaceuticals 51
molecular biology 24, 26, 48, 60
MONICA project 120
Monod 26
MORI 129, 130–1
Morris, J. 99
MRC's Operational and Ethical Guidelines
    on Human Tissue and Biological Samples
    for Use in Research (2001) 112
Mulderij, K. 89
Mulkay, M. 158, 168
Multi-centre Research Ethics Committees
    (MRECs) 112, 116
multi-gene paradigm 27
multifactorial conditions 33, 115
Murenberg 26
Murray, J. 87
Myriad Genetics 114, 117

National Health Service (NHS) 77, 107,
    137, 146, 148
National Human Genome Research
    Institute (NHGRI) 40–3, 50, 53, 56
National Institute of Health (NIH) 44, 53
National Screening Committee 66, 75,
    78, 147

nationhood 117–18
Nazis 20, 71, 106
Nelis, A. 29
Nelkin, D. 19, 25, 144
Nerlich, B. 156, 157, 158
Newman, S. 31
Newton, J. 116
Nicoll, A. 113
NINDS 56
non-directive counselling 33, 151
non-medical selection 32
non-statutory guidelines 29
normalization 89, 90, 91, 94, 95, 98–9
Novartis 129–30
Novas, C. 84, 85, 97–8
Nuffield Council on Bioethics 113, 148;
    Consultation on Genetic Screening 70
Nurse, Sir Paul 147

obesity 57
objectivity 15, 43, 131
obstetrician(s) 24, 27, 72
Office of Science and Technology 126, 128
One Stop Clinic for the Assessment of Risk
    (OSCAR) 75, 76
O'Neill, Baroness Onora 147
ownership 11, 28, 31, 46, 47, 51, 105,
    107, 118, 143, 144, 150, 166
Oxagen 104

Page, D. 109, 110, 111, 114
Pálsson, G. 120
Parens, E. 84, 99, 101
Parkinson's Disease Society 139
Parsons, E. 62, 81, 92, 132
past 1, 4, 5, 6, 7, 9, 10, 11, 13, 15–18, 21,
    25, 26, 27, 32, 34, 35, 37, 64, 71, 72,
    77, 82, 90, 105, 106, 121, 126, 136,
    143, 146, 149, 162–3, 165
Patent and Trademark Amendment Act
    (1980) 28
patenting 46, 48, 49, 62, 105, 107, 117,
    136, 147, 166
patents 2, 28, 46, 48–9, 54, 77, 107
patients 11, 13, 34, 36, 50, 73, 84–6, 101,
    106, 108, 113, 114, 120, 146, 160, 161,
    163–5, 166, 168; activists *see*
    campaigning organizations; groups 2,
    51–2, 53, 62, 107, 115, 118, 119, 138,
    147, 168; by proxy 12, 103, 110
Paul, D. 17, 20, 21, 23
Pelchart, D. 89
Penrose, L. 23

People Science and Policy Ltd. 115
perfection 143, 144
personalized medicine 145
Petersen, A. 71, 135, 157
pharmacogenomics 53
phenotype 27, 39, 60
Plenicar, M. 6
policy makers 13, 32, 50, 66, 142, 145–8
policy making 7, 36, 72, 80, 125, 134,
    135, 140, 153, 169
political economy 73, 107, 115, 117,
    131, 152
popular culture 3, 136
population policies 15, 18, 19
post-human futures 144, 149, 163
Poste, G. 116
pregnancy 24, 32, 34, 64, 66, 67, 70, 72,
    74, 75, 76, 77, 79, 81, 100, 103, 155,
    157, 168; *see also* reproduction
preimplantation genetic diagnosis (PGD)
    32, 65, 66, 67, 84
prenatal: diagnosis 66, 79, 84; screening
    65, 70, 72; testing 36, 65, 67, 80, 81,
    99, 101; tests 2, 67
present 4, 162–3
President's Council on Bioethics 149, 153
press release 12, 38, 39, 40–3, 44, 50, 53,
    56, 62, 159, 165
presymptomatic tests 2, 95
prevention of disease 3, 22–4, 33, 145,
    149, 155, 162
privacy and confidentiality 104, 106, 107,
    111–16
procreative autonomy 73
procreative beneficence 32
professional practice 7, 12, 13, 160,
    163, 167
professional standards 50
professionals 2, 3, 5, 7, 10, 11, 12, 13, 16,
    19, 20, 26, 32, 34–5, 36, 39, 50, 51, 52,
    53, 62, 66, 67, 73, 78, 79, 80, 82, 84,
    86, 88, 90, 92, 96, 97, 103, 105, 109,
    110, 113, 114, 116, 119, 120, 121, 131,
    132, 133, 136, 141, 144, 145, 146, 147,
    152, 154, 163–5
progress 5, 10, 13, 20, 30, 43, 56, 62, 65,
    71, 73, 103, 105, 111, 117, 120, 121,
    124, 144, 147, 151, 153, 156, 159, 160,
    162, 163, 166, 169
pseudo-science 17, 19
psychology 18, 19
psychosocial approach to health 11, 84, 85,
    86–9

Public Consultation on Developments in
    Biosciences (PCDB) 135
publics 7, 11, 50, 123–5, 160, 161, 163–5,
    168, 169; attitudes to science 126–7,
    130; consultation 105, 135;
    engagement 119, 120, 134, 136;
    health 12, 19, 23, 25, 27, 72, 73, 112,
    115; interest groups 109, 115, 136, 138;
    opinion 12, 123, 124, 125–32, 142;
    perception 4, 7; –private partnerships
    28, 104, 116; trust 7, 106, 107, 124,
    135; understanding of genetics 1, 3, 7,
    123–4, 129, 142; understanding of
    science, constructivist model 124, 132,
    134, 138
PXE International 118, 119

qualitative methods 134, 135, 136, 142
quantitative methods 134

Rabeharisoa, V. 51–2, 135
Rabinow, P. 5, 34, 51, 135–6
racial supremacy 15
Rapp, R. 66, 72, 80, 81, 84, 101, 168
reductionism 24–8, 148, 163
Reed, Sheldon 23
regulation(s) 3, 17, 29, 30, 48, 50, 57,
    131, 150, 151, 153, 157
Reilly, P. 109, 110, 111, 114
Reindal, S. 32
reproduction 10, 22, 32, 64–6
reproductive choice 13, 66–74, 78,
    79, 82
reproductive cloning 30, 146, 154, 160
reproductive genetics 6, 64, 65, 68, 70, 73,
    74, 82; screening 5, 11, 12, 64, 66, 83,
    123, 148, 167; technologies 10, 12, 64,
    66, 74, 166
research ethics 50, 53; committees 79, 106,
    108, 109, 117, 168
research funding 3, 43, 51, 54
research subjects, people as 12, 44, 89,
    95, 103, 108, 109, 110, 114, 116,
    123, 125, 134
Resnik, D. 154–5
responsibility 12, 18, 24, 30, 57, 65, 71,
    72, 76, 79, 81, 84, 85, 94, 95, 101, 107,
    120, 121, 133, 157, 162
Reynolds, T. 79
Richards, M. 84, 99, 100
Rifkin, J. 31, 151, 152
rights: individual 13, 162
Rimmer, M. 114

risk 2, 5, 6, 11, 13, 15, 22, 23, 25, 34, 35,
52, 65, 70, 73, 74, 75, 76, 80, 81, 84,
85, 86, 88, 90, 91, 92, 94–101, 105,
106, 109, 112, 113, 114, 119, 121, 126,
129, 131, 132, 133, 137, 143, 145, 149,
152, 154, 155, 156, 158, 161, 162, 164,
165; –benefit analysis 131, 155;
perception 133; reduction measures 92,
94, 95; society 5, 165
Roberts, C. 84
Roberts, L. 55
Rock, P. 17
Rommens, J. 58
Rose, H. 92, 132–3
Rose, N. 5, 22, 25, 36, 84, 85,
97–8, 144
Roslin Institute 50–1, 156–7
Rothman, B. 72, 81, 84
Rothstein, M. 35, 108
Royal Society, The 135, 136, 147
Ryley, H. 23

safety 77, 149, 153, 154, 156
Sainsbury, Lord 128
Sarkar, S. 26
Savulescu, J. 32, 70, 73
schizophrenia 33
Schutz 132
screening programmes *see* genetic
screening
Second World War 20, 73
Seed, R. 157
self-help groups 51
self-regulation 30
self-surveillance 22
Serum, Urine and Ultrasound Screening
Study (SURUSS) 77
service provision 6, 29, 54–5, 66, 75, 80,
82, 89, 148, 151, 152, 154
sex selection 65
Shakespeare, T. 10, 84, 99, 106
Shapiro, D. 79
Sharp, K. 71, 111, 119
Shepherd, M. 90
Shiloh, S. 23
Sibinga, M. 59
sickle-cell disease 84, 87, 99
Silver, L. 157
single gene disorders 2, 137
single nucleotide polymorphisms
(SNPs) 114
Smith, C. 5, 139
Social and Cultural Impact of the
New Genetics', 'The 12 n3, 174

social construction of genes 8, 9, 165
social control 17, 21, 27, 149, 162
social exclusion 22, 163
social order 8–9, 18
social progress 10, 13, 20, 103, 121, 124,
144, 162, 169
social research on genetics 1, 3, 4, 12, 13,
161–2, 164, 166, 167, 168, 169
social science 96, 167–8
somatic gene therapy 32–3
special interest groups *see* campaigning
organizations
Spencer, K. 75
Staley, K. 113, 115
standardization 47, 62, 82
Staples, S. 117
state, the 18, 28, 29–30, 31, 35, 45, 71,
72, 107, 124, 153
Stegmayr, B. 120
stem cell research 2, 31, 50–1, 52, 53,
139, 149, 150, 159
Stemerding, D. 66, 73, 75, 82
sterilization 17, 18–19, 20, 21, 22,
31–2, 71
Stewart, J. 136
stigma 35, 57, 80, 85, 88, 89, 100,
109, 162
Stock, G. 152–3, 154
Stockdale, A. 84, 98, 107
Sulston, J. 29
Super, M. 17
surveillance 18–22, 25, 57, 72, 81,
113, 115, 144

Taanila, L. 88
tailored medicine 2, 143, 145
Tanner, J. 88
Tauber, A. 26
technological determinism 153
termination *see* abortion
therapeutic cloning 146
Thomas, C. 99
Thomas, S. 29
Thompson, R. 87, 88
Thomson, Mark 19
'Transformations in Genetic Subjecthood'
12 n3, 69, 174
transparency 168
Trombley, S. 19, 21
trust 7, 12, 80, 106, 107–8, 110, 111–12,
119, 120, 121, 124, 133, 135, 137–8,
142, 158, 164
Tsui, L. 55–6
Turner, G. 133

UK Biobank 2, 104, 105, 115, 116
UK Biobank Industry Consultation Meeting
(2003) 116
UK Health and Social Care Act
(2001) 113
UK National Screening Committee:
Antenatal Subgroup 78, 79
UK Stem Cell Bank Steering
Committee 139
ultrasound screening 22, 64, 75, 76, 77
UNESCO's Universal Declaration on the
Human Genome and Human Rights
(1997) 30
US Department of Health and Human
Services 118
US Institutional Review Boards 112
US National Bioethics Advisory
Commission 109
US National Human Genome Research
Institute 114
US National Institutes of Health 118
US Patent and Trademarks Office
(PTO) 118

Van Dijck, J. 26, 38, 157–8, 159
Venter, C. 46, 49
Verity, C. 113
Ville, I. 98
voluntarism 18–22, 27

Wald, N. 24, 74, 75, 77, 78
Waldby, C. 47
Walsh, V. 46–7
Warner, M. 123, 124
Watson, J. 21
Webster, A. 4, 29
Weinberg, D. 39
Weismann 25
welfare 18, 19, 21, 71, 112
Wellcome Trust, The 3, 126, 128, 136,
174,
Welsh Citizens' Jury 137
Welsh Institute for Health and Social
Care 137
Werdnig-Hoffman syndrome 99, 100
Whittle, M. 74, 78
Wieting, S. 116, 117
Williams, C. 5, 66, 72, 74, 79, 158, 159
Williams, G. 85
Williamson, R. 55
Winston, R. 65
Woolgar, S. 161
World Health Organization (WHO)
*Proposed International Guidelines on
Ethical Issues in Medical Genetics and
Genetic Services* (1998) 30
World Medical Association 111–12
Wright, S. 28
Wynne, B. 124, 128, 129, 132, 133, 141

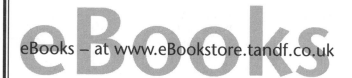